VOICES FROM THE ETHER

The History of Radio

By

Gordon Bathgate

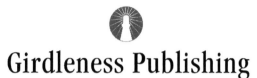

Girdleness Publishing

49 Girdleness Road
Torry, Aberdeen,
Scotland,
AB11 8DG
Telephone: 01224 891106
Email: girdlenessbooks@aol.com

ISBN 978-1-4716-2861-0

Contents

1) Prologue   Page 4

2) The Fathers of Radio   Page 5

3) The British Broadcasting Company   Page 24

4) The British Broadcasting Corporation   Page 50

5) Radio in America   Page 62

6) Voices from Europe   Page 81

7) Radio at War   Page 95

8) The End of the Golden Age   Page 115

9) Radio Down Under   Page 125

10) Radio Fights Back   Page 137

11) Radio in the 21st Century   Page 155

12) Bibliography   Page 166

1
Prologue

As a small child I remember being fascinated by the large wooden box that sat in the corner of our living room. I'd watch intently as one of my parents switched it on and a warm yellow glow would radiate from the panel on the front. I loved to hear the strange whistling, whooshing, squeaking, crackling and popping noises that emanated from the box as either my mother or father twiddled the knob until some music filled the room.

I soon learned how to work the box myself and would twiddle the knob feverishly to hear that strange cacophony of noise at every opportunity, much to the annoyance of my parents. Luckily for them, I swiftly tired of the discordant racket and discovered that if I tuned around the dial slowly I could hear more. I would tune around until I heard a voice or piece of music. It didn't matter what it was, I'd sit quietly listening to the ghostly voices from the ether pervading around the room.

This early fascination for radio has stayed with me throughout my life and I suspect I'll be listening to it when I'm in my dotage. So my lifelong passion has led me to the point where I had to write this book. I've delved deep into the history of radio's development and turned the spotlight on the innovators who helped make it possible. This book also features the personalities and programmes that have helped shape radio's destiny. I also examine the current media landscape and attempt to predict what the future holds for radio.

This book is dedicated to James Clerk Maxwell, Heinrich Hertz and Guglielmo Marconi. Thanks for inventing this crazy thing called radio guys - it's given me a lifetime of pleasure and happiness.

2

The Fathers Of Radio

In the late 19th century it was clear to numerous scientists that wireless communication was possible. Various theoretical and experimental advancements led to the development of radio and the communication system we know today. The key invention for the beginning of 'wireless transmission of data using the entire frequency spectrum' was the spark-gap transmitter. These devices served as the transmitters for most wireless telegraphy systems for the first three decades of radio.

During its early development, and long after widespread use of the technology, disputes persisted as to the person who could claim sole credit for the invention of radio. Many experiments were running concurrently and across continents. Some scientific theories were merely notional and later proved unworkable but they also helped fuel other ideas that did advance technology.

There are several men who have been proclaimed the 'father of radio' but perhaps one simple way to sort out the parentage is to place events in a rough chronological order.

The hypothesis that electricity and magnetism, both capable of causing attraction and repulsion of objects, were linked was proposed by various scientists. In 1802, Gian Domenico Romagnosi proposed the relationship between electric current and magnetism, but his reports were largely ignored. In 1820, Hans Christian Ørsted conducted a widely known experiment on man-made electric current and magnetism. He established that a wire carrying a current could deflect a magnetized compass needle. Ørsted's experiments discovered the relationship between electricity and magnetism in a very simple experiment. Ørsted's work influenced André-Marie Ampère's theory of electromagnetism.

The British physicist Michael Faraday had discovered the existence of the electro-magnetic fields in 1845. Michael Faraday, the son of a blacksmith, was born in London in 1791. He was apprenticed to a bookbinder and this contact with books gave him a love of reading. After becoming interested in science, Faraday applied to Humphrey Davy for a job.

Davy gave Faraday a valuable scientific education and also introduced him to important scientists in Europe. Faraday's greatest contribution to science was in the field of electricity. In 1831, Michael Faraday began a series of experiments in which he discovered electromagnetic induction. Faraday developed the theory that a current flowing in one wire could induce a current in another wire that was not physically connected to the first. Although Faraday was the first to publish his results, the American scientist Joseph Henry had also been working on a similar theory.

James Clerk Maxwell, the Scottish physicist, was born on June 13th 1831, in Edinburgh. He was fascinated by Faraday and Henry's work on electromagnetism. He noticed that electrical fields and magnetic fields could couple together to form electromagnetic waves. Neither an electrical field (like the static which forms when you rub your feet on a carpet), nor a magnetic field (like the one that holds a magnet onto your refrigerator) will go anywhere by themselves. But, Maxwell discovered that a varying magnetic field would induce a varying electric field and vice-versa.

An electromagnetic wave exists when the changing magnetic field causes a changing electric field, which then causes another changing magnetic field, and so on forever. Unlike a static field, a wave cannot exist unless it is moving. Once produced, an electromagnetic wave will carry on forever unless matter absorbs it.

In 1864 Maxwell published his first paper that showed by theoretical reasoning that an electrical disturbance resulting from a change in an electrical quantity, such as voltage or current, should propagate through space at the speed of light. Maxwell finally published this work in his 'Treatise on Electricity and Magnetism' in 1873.

In 1866, a dentist from Washington DC called Dr Mahlon Loomis described a system of signalling by radio. Dr Loomis claimed to have transmitted signals between two Blue Ridge Mountain-tops 14 miles apart in Virginia, using two kites as antennas. The kites had 600ft wires attacked to them. Both ends were grounded; one through a galvanometer. When he disconnected and reconnected one end, the amount of current flowing through the other end changed. He therefore claims to be the first person to achieve wireless, electronic communication.

Mahlon Loomis received U.S. Patent 129,971 for a 'wireless telegraph' in July 1872. This patent utilizes atmospheric electricity to eliminate the overhead wire used by the existing telegraph systems. It did not contain diagrams or specific methods and it did not refer to or incorporate any known scientific theory. It is substantially similar to William Henry Ward's patent that was issued a few months earlier. Neither patent referred to any known scientific theory of electromagnetism and could never have received and transmitted radio waves. It's widely assumed that Loomis exaggerated his achievements to sustain interest in a system that he undoubtedly believed would work.

Towards the end of 1875, while experimenting with the telegraph, Thomas Edison noted a phenomenon that he termed 'etheric force', announcing it to the press on the 28th November. He abandoned this research when Elihu Thomson, among others, ridiculed the idea. The idea was not based on the electromagnetic waves described by Maxwell.

In 1878, David E. Hughes was the first to claim to have transmitted and received radio waves when he noticed that his induction balance caused noise in the receiver of his homemade telephone. He demonstrated his discovery to the Royal Society in 1880 but was told it was merely induction. Hughes was so disheartened he didn't publish the results of his work. Although he continued experimenting with radio, it was left to others to document his findings and by that time radio had passed him by.

In 1884, the Italian Temistocle Calzecchi-Onesti demonstrated a primitive device that would later be developed to become the first practical radio detector. By placing metal filings in a glass box or tube, and making them part of an ordinary electric circuit.

In 1890, Edouard Branly of France demonstrated a much improved version of Calzecchi-Onesti's device. He called his version a "radio-conductor' but it would later be known as a 'coherer'. Branly demonstrated that such a tube would respond to sparks produced at a distance from it.

In 1885, Edison took out U.S. Patent 465,971 on a system of radio communication between ships. The patent, however, was not based on the transmission and reception of electromagnetic waves. He later sold the patent to Marconi.

James Clerk Maxwell's theoretical prediction that electromagnetic waves travel at the speed of light was verified in 1888. German physicist Heinrich Hertz made the amazing discovery of radio waves, a type of electromagnetic radiation with wavelengths too long for our eyes to see. He demonstrated the transmission and reception of the electromagnetic waves predicted by Maxwell and thus was the first person to intentionally transmit and receive radio.

Hertz created a transmitting oscillator, which radiated radio waves, and detected them using a metal loop with a gap at one side. When the loop was placed within the transmitter's electromagnetic field, sparks were produced across the gap. Hertz showed in his experiments that these signals possessed all of the properties of electromagnetic waves.

With this oscillator, Hertz solved two problems. The first was timing Maxwell's waves. He had physically demonstrated what Maxwell had only theorized - that the velocity of radio waves was equal to the velocity of light. This proved that radio waves were a form of light. Second, Hertz found out how to make the electric and magnetic fields detach themselves from wires and go free as Maxwell's waves. These waves became known as 'Hertzian Waves' and Hertz managed to detect them across the length of his laboratory. Famously, he saw no practical use for his discovery.

Nikola Tesla, a Serbian-American inventor began his research into radio in 1891. Two years later, Tesla gave a public demonstration of 'wireless' radio communication. Addressing the Franklin Institute in Philadelphia he described in detail the principles of radio communication.

Tesla's contribution involved refining and improving the technology developed by his predecessors. A most important innovation was the introduction of the coupled tuned circuit into his preliminary transmitter design. This was the Tesla Coil; with its primary and secondary circuits both synchronised to vibrate together in harmony.

The apparatus that Tesla used contained all the elements that were incorporated into radio systems before the development of the early vacuum tube, known then as an oscillation valve. Tesla initially used sensitive electromagnetic receivers, which were unlike the less responsive coherers later used by Marconi and other early experimenters.

Further modifications resulted in a transmitter that could have signalled across the Atlantic, had such an endeavour been made. Supplementary work resulted in the development of wireless receivers that also included two synchronized circuits.

Afterward, the principle of radio communication was publicized widely from Tesla's experiments and demonstrations. Various scientists, inventors, and experimenters began to investigate wireless methods.

Claims have been made that Nathan B. Stubblefield, an eccentric farmer from Murray, Kentucky developed radio between 1885 and 1892, before either Tesla or Marconi. Stubblefield was convinced other people were stealing his ideas but his devices seemed to have worked by induction transmission rather than radio transmission.

Nathan B. Stubblefield died of starvation in 1928. The citizens of Murray, Kentucky, were highly affectionate towards their mad radio genius. They called him 'The Father of Radio' and erected a monument to him in the town in 1930.

Between 1893 and 1894, Roberto Landell de Moura, a Brazilian priest and scientist, conducted experiments in wireless transmissions. He didn't publicize his achievement until 1900, when he held a public demonstration of a wireless transmission of voice in São Paulo, Brazil on June 3. He was granted a Brazilian patent in 1901 before securing three more for a Wave Transmitter, a Wireless Telephone and Wireless Telegraph. However these inventions failed to develop further due to lack of funding.

In November 1894, the Indian physicist, Jagdish Chandra Bose, demonstrated publicly the use of radio waves in Calcutta. Bose ignited gunpowder and rang a bell at a distance using electromagnetic waves, proving that communication signals can be sent without using wires. He was therefore the first to send and receive radio waves over a significant distance. Bose didn't commercially exploit this achievement as he wasn't interested in patenting his work.

The public demonstration by Bose in Calcutta was before Marconi's wireless signalling experiment on Salisbury Plain in England in May 1897. In 1896, the English Daily Chronicle reported on his UHF experiments:

"The inventor (J.C. Bose) has transmitted signals to a distance of nearly a mile and herein lies the first and obvious and exceedingly valuable application of this new theoretical marvel."

Oliver Lodge transmitted radio signals on August 14, 1894 at a meeting of the British Association for the Advancement of Science at Oxford University. This was one year after Tesla, five years after Heinrich Hertz and one year before Marconi. On 19th August 1894, Lodge demonstrated the reception of Morse code signalling via radio waves using a coherer. He improved Edouard Branly's coherer radio wave detector by adding a trembler which dislodged clumped filings, thus restoring the device's sensitivity. In August 1898 he got U.S. Patent 609,154, 'Electric Telegraphy' that made wireless signals using Ruhmkorff coils or Tesla coils for the transmitter and a Branly coherer for the detector. This was a key factor in the 'syntonic' tuning concept developed later by Marconi. In fact Lodge sold the patent to Marconi in 1912.

In 1895, the physicist Alexander Popov developed a practical communication system based on the coherer. His invention was capable of detecting electromagnetic waves that indicated the presence of electrical discharges, specifically lightning, in the atmosphere. The design of Popov's lightning detector was similar to that of Marconi's wireless telegraph, but Popov's invention focused on receiving rather than transmitting signals. He didn't apply for a patent for this invention.

Popov had extrapolated upon the work of earlier physicists, namely Heinrich Hertz and Oliver Lodge, but Popov's was the first to incorporate an antenna. Another significant discovery of Popov's came in 1897, when he found that metallic objects could interfere with the transmission of radio waves, a phenomenon known as wave reflection.

On May 7th 1895, Popov performed a public demonstration of transmission and reception of radio waves used for communication at the Russian Physical and Chemical Society Popov's early experiments were transmissions of only 600 yards Around March 1896, Popov demonstrated in public the transmission of radio waves, between different campus buildings to the Saint Petersburg Physical Society. This was before the public demonstration of the Marconi system.

However other accounts state that Popov achieved these results only in December 1897 after publication of Marconi's patent. Later Popov experimented with ship-to-shore communication. Popov died in 1905 and his claim was not pressed by the Russian government until 1945.

In 1895, The New Zealander Ernest Rutherford arrived in England with a reputation as an innovator and inventor. The 1st Baron Rutherford of Nelson distinguished himself in several fields, initially by working out the electrical properties of solids and then using wireless waves as a method of signalling. Rutherford was encouraged in his work by Sir Robert Ball, who had been scientific adviser to the body maintaining lighthouses on the Irish coast. he wished to solve the difficult problem of a ship's inability to detect a lighthouse in fog. Sensing fame and fortune, Rutherford increased the sensitivity of his apparatus until he could detect electromagnetic waves over a distance of several hundred metres. The commercial development, though, of wireless technology was left for others, as Rutherford continued purely scientific research.

Karl Ferdinand Braun made two major contributions to the development of radio. The first was the introduction of a closed tuned circuit in the generating part of the transmitter, and its separation from the antenna by means of inductive coupling. Around 1898, he invented a crystal diode rectifier or Cat's whisker diode. Braun's invention bridged a much longer distance.

Italian born Guglielmo Marconi was fascinated by Heinrich Hertz's discovery of radio waves, and realised that if they could be transmitted and detected over long distances, wireless telegraphy could be developed. He started experimenting in 1894 and set up rough aerials on opposite sides of the family garden. His aerials were tin plates mounted on posts. He managed to receive signals over a distance of 100 metres, and by the end of 1895 had extended the distance to over a mile. Marconi offered his telegraph system to the Italian Government, but they turned it down.

The British Post Office was more receptive and Marconi moved to London in 1896. In February he set up his transmitter on the roof of the Central Telegraph Office, and a receiver on the roof of a building called 'GPO South' in Carter Lane, 300 yards away. His later transmissions were detected 1.5 miles away, and on 2nd September at Salisbury plain the range was increased to 8 miles.

Marconi received the first wireless patent from the British Government. In part, it was based on the theory that communication range increases substantially as the height of the aerial above ground level increases. On December 12th 1896, Marconi gave his first public demonstration of radio at Toynbee Hall, London.

In 1897 Marconi established the Wireless Telegraph and Signal Company at Chelmsford. The world's first radio factory was opened there employing fifty people. On 11th May 1897 tests were carried out to establish that contacts were possible over water. A transmitter was set up at Lavernock Point, near Penarth and the transmissions were received on the other side of the Bristol Channel at the Island of Holm, a distance of 3.5 miles

In November 1897, the first permanent radio installation 'Needles Hotel Wireless Station' was installed at Alum Bay, Isle of Wight by the Wireless Telegraph and Signal Company. Alum Bay was an isolated but striking strip of coastline that provided open water straight to the mainland just as far as his equipment's top range.

Marconi established his first radio station in sight of the famous 'Needles', where he managed to transmit to two hired ferryboats and another station in Bournemouth. Alum Bay may have helped launch wireless but this didn't impress the inventor's landlord, the Royal Needles Hotel, which raised his rent. Marconi's dismantled the station at the end of May 1900 and moved further down the coast.

The Daily Express was the first newspaper to obtain news by wireless telegraphy in August 1898. In December 1898 Marconi set up radio equipment on the Royal Yacht Osbourne, which was moored at Cowes, Isle of Wight. Regular messages were relayed from the yacht and Osborne House, also in the Isle of Wight. The messages were then passed on to Buckingham Palace. The Queen received 150 bulletins on the Prince of Wales' health, by radio, from the yacht, where he was convalescing. The Prince operated the equipment on the Royal Yacht while Marconi operated the equipment in Osbourne house. Around the same time, wireless communication was set up between the East Goodwin light ship and the South Foreland lighthouse.

In 1899 Captain Jackson, on board the HMS Defiant (an old wooden battle ship which had been converted into a Royal Navy torpedo school) gave orders to three cruisers in controlled manoeuvres, via radio for the first time. Marconi was on board as an observer. The first telegraph message was sent across the English Channel on March 27th 1899. It was sent from South Foreland to Wimereux, in France by Marconi. The success of the demonstration resulted in lighthouses throughout the UK being fitted with wireless sets.

On 17th March 1899, Marconi obtained a lot of publicity when the first life was saved by wireless telegraphy, which was used to save a ship in distress in the North Sea. The three masted ship 'Elbe' was sailing to Hamburg with a cargo of slates. It went ashore on the Goodwin Sands at 2 in the morning; a thick fog was prevailing at the time. The East Goodwin Lightship heard the signals and communicated by wireless telegraphy to the South Foreland Lighthouse. From there telegraphic messages were sent to the authorities. The lifeboats at Ramsgate, Deal, and Kingsdown were put on standby. Fortunately the lifeboats weren't required as the 'Elbe' was able to re-float eight hours later. Nevertheless this was the first occasion in the history of the world in which lifeboats had been alerted by the means of wireless.

About this time Marconi began to develop tuned circuits for wireless transmission, so that a wireless can be tuned to a particular frequency. He patented this on 26th April 1900, under the name of 'Tuned Syntonic Telegraphy'.

Marconi's next project was to send a signal across the Atlantic. He convinced investors to spend £50,000 on the transatlantic project Marconi purchased land in Poldhu, Cornwall. Poldhu was chosen by Marconi because it stood directly opposite Cap Cod, where its sister radio station was to be built. The site was also chosen for its remoteness to keep the project out of the public eye and out of the newspapers.

It was a massive undertaking, which dwarfed anything he had built before. Construction work began in October 1900. Around 400 wires were suspended in an inverted cone shape from twenty 200ft high masts. Infuriatingly the system was blown down during a storm, so a temporary aerial was hastily set up, using two surviving masts, to let the transatlantic experiments carry on. A year later, the Poldhu Wireless Station had successfully transmitted wireless signals to ships at distances over 200 miles. However the Transatlantic project remained Marconi's main goal.

On the other side of the Atlantic, the Cape Cod site was eventually abandoned. Numerous difficulties including severe weather necessitated the move of the receiving station from Cape Cod to St. John's Newfoundland, which was also 600 miles closer to Cornwall.

Marconi travelled across the Atlantic to supervise proceedings from that end. Due to time and financial constraints, he opted not to build a masted receiving antenna array. The original receiving antenna in Newfoundland was four inches in diameter and was held aloft by a balloon, which was ripped apart in a storm. The first attempt to send signals across was made in November 1901. The test failed when one of 2 balloons holding 600 feet of aerial wire broke it's mooring and floated away.

At 12:30 a.m. on December 12, 1901, at Signal Hill in St. John's Newfoundland, Marconi heard three faint clicks through the earphones of his wireless receiver - the Morse code letter 'S' -and a new era was born. The receiving aerial, 600 feet of wire, was held aloft by 6 kites flying at an altitude of 400 feet.

The British Government and Admiralty were greatly impressed and many people wanted to invest in the new technology. The Government assumed control of the station at Poldhu during the First World War. It eventually closed down in 1933. A small museum stands on the site now.

Demand grew and large numbers of ships carried the new apparatus, which saved many lives at sea. One of the most famous occasions was when the Titanic sank. Titanic's wireless set had a nominal working range of 250 nautical miles, but signalling more distant stations was possible. At night, ranges of up to 2,000 miles were attained with sets of similar design. The 'T' type aerial that was used offered greater power and sensitivity, both fore and aft. Therefore optimised performance could be expected when the ship was pointed either toward or away from a distant station. The ability to send signals over great distances helped to summon assistance much quicker and undoubtedly saved many lives.

The aspirations of the early radio pioneers did not include the broadcasting of music and information into homes using wireless. However some people saw it as a serious wireless alternative to the Bell telephone.

Conveying voice or music by radio required a continuous-wave transmitter. In 1902, Danish engineer Valdemar Poulsen invented an arc converter as a generator of continuous-wave radio signals. Beginning in 1904, Poulsen used the arc for experimental radio communication from Lyngby to various sites in Denmark and Great Britain.

The radiotelephone years, 1900-1920, were known more for the rival voice transmission technologies than for broadcasting. While spark was quickly rejected as too noisy and the alternator as too costly, it was the many versions of the Poulsen arc that clearly dominated radiotelephone inventions and early broadcasting for an audience

Marconi saw no need for voice transmission. He felt that the Morse code was adequate for communication between ships and across oceans. Marconi didn't anticipate the development of the radio and broadcasting industry and he left the early experimentation with wireless telephony to others.

Professor Reginald Aubrey Fessenden's technology and circuit arrangements were very different to Marconi's. He tried all the various methods of generating wireless signals in the early days, by spark, by arc and by the high frequency alternator. His work was dominated by his interest in transmitting words without wires. Fessenden's equipment included a spark transmitter, using a Wehnelt interrupter working a Ruhmkorff induction coil. In 1899 he noted, when the key was held down for a long dash, that the odd wailing sound of the Wehnelt interrupter could be clearly heard in the receiving telephone. This suggested to him that by using a spark rate far above voice band, wireless telephony could be achieved.

On the 23rd December he succeeded in transmitting speech over a distance of 1.5 km. By 1904 fairly satisfactory speech had been transmitted by the arc method. Nevertheless Fessenden was an advocate of the continuous wave method of wireless transmission.

He developed his new high frequency alternator-transmitter showing its utility for point-to-point wireless telephony, including interconnecting his stations to the wire telephone network. Fessenden placed a carbon microphone directly in line between his alternator and the antenna lead.

Fessenden also invented the heterodyne effect. In this, a received radio wave is combined with a wave of a frequency slightly different from the carrier wave. The intermediate frequency wave that is produced as a result is easier to amplify, and can then be demodulated to generate the original sound wave.

Marconi's transatlantic experiments had captured the public's imagination. Fessenden had also been conducting his own transatlantic experiments from the National Electric Signalling Company at Brant Rock in Massachusetts.

To carry out transatlantic transmission experiments Fessenden's Company built a station at Machrihanish in Scotland, installing equipment the duplicate of that at Brant Rock. After numerous attempts it became evident that no signals were coming through from Scotland. Fessenden sent his best engineer, Mr. Armor, to Scotland. The reply came in January 1906. Armor sent a telegram saying that Machrihanish was receiving the signals from Massachusetts loud and clear.

Encouraged by this achievement, Fessenden enhanced the effectiveness of his high frequency alternator and with a new type of umbrella antenna of his own design; both stations were in regular communication. In June a small testing station had been built at Plymouth, eleven miles from Brant Rock. The engineers used voice transmission to communicate with each other.

In November a letter was received from Mr. Armor containing the astounding news that he had clearly heard the complete conversation of Mr. Stein at Brant Rock telling the operator at Plymouth "how to run the dynamo". Therefore the first human voice to be transmitted across the Atlantic was that of Mr. Stein.

The Machrihanish tower collapsed during a severe winter storm on 5th December 1906. The station was never rebuilt, and so Fessenden's transatlantic trials came to a rapid conclusion. Instead he decided to concentrate on developing voice transmission.

On Christmas Eve, 1906, from his workshop in Chestnut Hill, Massachusetts, Fessenden sent a Morse message alerting all ships at sea to expect an important transmission. What they heard that night was the first public broadcast of the human voice.

Fessenden gave a brief description of the forthcoming broadcast then played an Edison wax-cylinder recording of Handel's Largo. Fessenden then treated his listeners to his rendition of 'Oh Holy Night' on the violin and actually singing the last verse as he played. Fessenden's wife Helen and his secretary Miss Bent had promised to read passages from the Bible. However when the time came to perform they froze and Fessenden took over for them. Fessenden concluded the broadcast by extending Christmas greetings to his listeners and asked them to write and report to him on the broadcast wherever they were. The broadcast was successfully repeated on New Year's Eve.

Fessenden's methods were extremely primitive when compared to today's standards. They were, however, the first real departure from Marconi's damped-wave-coherer system for telegraphy, which other experimenters were merely emulating or adapting. They were the first ground breaking steps toward radio communications and radio broadcasting.

In 1907 The British Admiralty authorised Lieutenant Quentin Crawford to set up an experimental radio station on board HMS Andromeda. Using the call sign QFP, he adapted the spark wireless transmitter on board to broadcast a programme featuring music and speech for the benefit of the Royal Navy fleet in Chatham dockyard. Crawford's historic inaugural broadcast was a patriotic concert program performed by navy personnel.

Harry Grindell Matthews was a British wireless experimenter who demonstrated the versatility of wireless telephony by being the first to communicate with a moving aircraft. On Saturday, September 23rd 1911 at Ely Racecourse in Cardiff, Matthews established radio contact with C.B. Hucks, an aeronautical pilot, flying at a height of 700 feet and at a speed of 60 miles per hour. Some years later, Matthews claimed to have perfected a way of transmitting energy without wires. He claimed that his 'Death Ray' would be able to shoot down aeroplanes and explode ammunition dumps.

In 1904, Sir John Ambrose Fleming invented the thermionic diode or valve, which assisted the detection of high-frequency radio waves. He'd adapted Edison's electric lamp and added a second element called a plate. His invention was a major step forward in wireless technology as it was considerably more efficient as a radio wave detector than coherers or magnetic detectors. Valves became fundamental components in radios, as well as television sets and computers for 50 years, before being superseded by the transistor.

In January 1907, American Lee De Forest patented the triode valve, which he called the 'audion'. De Forest modified Ambrose Fleming's design by adding a grid to control and amplify radio and sound waves.

Later that year he formed the De Forest Radio Telephone Company and began seeking investors. As De Forest (and hundreds of other inventors) unfortunately discovered, you had to be a promoter as well as an inventor. Arguably, there was no wireless and radio inventor who was associated by more controversy than Lee de Forest. He was occasionally linked with unsavoury business promoters and was accused frequently of dishonest business practices. He fought for decades to persuade the scientific community that he deserved to be known as the 'Father of Radio'. De Forest spent millions in court battles trying to validate and re-validate his patents.

People's opinions are divided about De Forest. He seems to be vilified or sanctified in equal measure. However the evidence robustly indicates that Lee de Forest was the first to want to use the wireless for more than two-way commercial message traffic.

De Forest was a music lover and in an early company article, he predicted, "It will soon be possible to distribute grand opera music from transmitters placed on the stage of the Metropolitan Opera House by a Radio Telephone station on the roof to almost any dwelling in Greater New York and vicinity".

That prediction eventually happened on January 12, 1910. De Forest conducted an experimental broadcast of the live performance of the opera Tosca. The next day, he broadcast a performance with the participation of the Italian tenor Enrico Caruso. The audiences for these broadcasts were largely journalists who were invited to experience the events. They were huddled round receivers placed strategically in different parts of New York.

By the start of 1916, De Forest had refined his audion to be used as an oscillator for the radiotelephone. He sold it to the telephone company as an amplifier of transcontinental phone calls.

Later that year, De Forest, broadcast the first radio advertisements from experimental radio station 2XG in New York City. The advertisements were for his own products incidentally. De Forest went on to sponsor radio broadcasts of music but he received little financial backing.

He also transmitted the first Presidential election report by radio in November 1916. He broadcast from his station in The Bronx, New York assisted by a wire supplied by the Republican newspaper 'The New York American'. De Forest sent bulletins out every hour. Between the bulletins listeners heard The Star-Spangled Banner and other anthems, songs, and hymns. The broadcast lasted approximately six hours until signing off about 11 p.m. Unfortunately De Forest ended his broadcast before Woodrow Wilson came from behind to win. So many of the listeners heard the wrong candidate declared the winner.

A few months later, De Forest moved his tube transmitter to High Bridge, New York. He had been granted a licence from the Department of Commerce for an experimental radio station, but had to cease all broadcasting when the U.S. entered World War I in April 1917.

De Forest resumed his broadcasts from High Bridge, New York after the war but fell foul of the U.S Federal Inspector. He moved his operations to California in April 1920. De Forest operated his station 6XC from the California Theatre until November 1921. The transmitter was moved to Oakland and 6XC became KZY, the Rock Ridge Station.

Lee De Forest moved on to work on a variety of non-radio technical devices, most notably his Phonofilm system, a process to make the movies talk by adding a synchronized optical soundtrack to the film.

In his final years De Forest was disillusioned at what radio programming had become. Speaking to reporters he asked, "Why should anyone want to buy a radio? Nine tenths of what one can hear is the continual drivel of second-rate jazz, sickening crooning by degenerate sax players, interrupted by blatant sales talks"

Before the First World War, receivers were mainly crystal sets, which were exceedingly insensitive and unselective. They were connected to a pair of headphones and required a long aerial. In Britain, the new technology was strictly controlled by the Post Office. It was reasonably simple to acquire a receiving licence but a much more complicated proposition to obtain permission to use a transmitter.

The Post Office had to be satisfied that the applicant had suitable engineering qualifications, or knowledge, to operate the transmitter. Transmitter output power was restricted to ten watts, and use was only permitted for scientific research or for something of use to the public. Only a small number of radio amateurs were transmitting before the First World War.

Like many other wars, the First World War hastened the development of technology that was useful for the war effort. Although valves had been produced since 1904, the inability to produce a good vacuum meant that these devices were unreliable and had a short life.

Irving Langmuir was an American scientist, best known to the electrical industry as the inventor of the gas filled tungsten lamp. Langmuir developed a method of producing an excellent vacuum. His first major development was the improvement of the diffusion pump, which ultimately led to the invention of the high-vacuum tube.

French military scientists used Langmuir's technique to produce a reliable and efficient triode valve, which was called the 'R' valve. It was used in military communication equipment and was produced in large numbers. After 1916, lamp manufacturers Osram, BTH also produced the valve in England.

When the war ended, many of these valves appeared on the surplus market and so were readily obtainable. A lot of people were interested in the new technology and began building receivers so the number of radio amateurs grew rapidly. The new valves made it possible to easily transmit high quality speech and music, and allowed high sensitivity receivers to be developed.

The first regularly scheduled broadcasts had begun in America in 1912. Charles D. Herrold, known as Doc, was working at a San Francisco wireless company as a Chief Engineer. He had lost everything he had when the 1906 earthquake struck. He fled San Francisco after the earthquake but when he returned in 1909, he opened his own school - The Herrold College of Wireless and Engineering. By all accounts he was an excellent teacher. His spare time was spent inventing ways to make his wireless radio inventions talk.

Charles Herrold did not claim to be the first to transmit the human voice but he claimed to be the first to conduct 'broadcasting'. He coined the terms 'narrowcasting' and 'broadcasting', respectively to identify transmissions destined for a single receiver such as that on board a ship, and those transmissions destined for a general audience. Herrold was the son of a Santa Clara Valley farmer and the term 'broadcasting' was originally a farming idiom meaning to spread seed over a large expanse.

To help the radio signal to spread in all directions, he designed some omnidirectional antennas, which he mounted on the rooftops of various buildings in San Jose. Herrold also claims to be the first broadcaster to accept advertising. He exchanged publicity for a local record store for records to play on his station.

Herrold made the first planned radio broadcast from his radio school. His station used spark-gap technology, but modulated the carrier frequency with the human voice, and later music. The station 'San Jose Calling' (there were no call letters), continued to eventually become KCBS in San Francisco.

However, Herrold did not profit financially from his pioneering work, and later became a repair technician and a janitor. He died in a Californian rest home, aged 72.

American Edwin Armstrong invented three of the basic electronic circuits underlying all modern radio, radar, and television. In 1914, while still an undergraduate, he patented the regenerative circuit, the superheterodyne receiver (1918) and the super-regenerative circuit in 1922.

Many of Armstrong's inventions were ultimately claimed by others in patent lawsuits. In particular, the regenerative circuit, which Armstrong patented in 1914 as a 'wireless receiving system,' was patented by Lee De Forest two years later. De Forest then sold the rights of his patent to AT&T.

Between 1922 and 1934, Armstrong found himself embroiled in a patent war. On one side were Armstrong, RCA, and Westinghouse, and De Forest and AT&T on the other. This action was the longest patent lawsuit ever litigated up to that period. Armstrong won the first round of the lawsuit, lost the second, and the third ended in stalemate. Ultimately De Forest was granted the regeneration patent at the Supreme Court of the United States. Many people today believe this result was due to a misunderstanding of the technical facts.

While the regenerative-circuit lawsuit dragged on, Armstrong was already working on another significant invention. He created wide-band frequency modulation radio or FM. Rather than varying the amplitude of a radio wave to create sound; Armstrong's method varied the frequency of the wave instead. FM radio broadcasts delivered a much clearer sound, free of static, than the AM radio dominant at the time.

However in the depressed 1930s the radio industry was in no mood to take on a new system that required a radical overhaul of both transmitters and receivers. Armstrong found himself boxed in on every side. It took him until 1940 to get a permit for the first FM station, erected at his own expense, on the Hudson River Palisades at Alpine, New Jersey. It would be another two years before the Federal Communications Commission allocated him a few frequencies.

After a hiatus caused by World War II, FM broadcasting began to expand. Armstrong again found himself impeded by the FCC, which ordered FM into a new frequency band at limited power. In addition, he had been immersed in litigation by a coterie of corporations on the basic rights to his invention and this left him financially drained and feeling depressed.

Armstrong was unable to face another long legal battle. On the night of January 31st 1954, dressed in his coat and hat, Armstrong jumped to his death from the thirteenth floor window of his New York City apartment. His suicide note to his wife said: "May God help you and have mercy on my soul". His widow Marion renewed the patent fight and ultimately won some $10 million in damages.

In 1947, three research physicists working at Bell Laboratories in America developed the transistor. Walter Brattain, John Bardeen and William Shockley realised that pioneering research into crystals carried out by Russell Ohl a decade earlier could lead to a solid-state alternative to the thermionic valve. The transistor was smaller and more reliable than its cumbersome predecessor. This meant that radios could become smaller and more portable.

The first transistor radio to be produced commercially went on sale in November 1954. The Regency TR-1 operated from a 22.5-volt battery and sold for $49.95. Sadly the high price meant that sales were poor initially. However within a few years prices had fallen sufficiently and transistor radios became very popular.

The birth of radio was a long drawn out affair. It had a disparate group of inventors and entrepreneurs all claiming parentage but we are no nearer to finding one single person who could claim to be the 'father of radio'.

These men had the marvellous gift to develop their own inventions or adapt other people's theories and ideas. Together they created a marvellous piece of technology that helped to save lives and influence and entertain others.

By the early 1920s, radio had advanced sufficiently from an invention that was the exclusive preserve of hobbyists and enthusiasts to a medium with real mass-market appeal. Radio was about to hit the mainstream.

3

The British Broadcasting Company

After the First World War, British wireless experimenters, or 'hams', moved away from Morse code transmissions and began to use wireless telephony. At one point nearly twenty stations were transmitting speech and music to the London area on Sunday mornings.

Some of the broadcasters included Harry Walker (2OM) who always introduced his musical programmes with 'This is Brentford Calling!' Bill Corsham (2UV) also gave local talent the opportunity to broadcast. He is also credited as the inventor of the QSL card. He would reply to anyone who sent a reception report by sending a card confirming details of the broadcast.

People quickly realised the potential for the commercial broadcasting of speech and music. Early in 1920, the Marconi Company began test transmissions from their Chelmsford base. These transmissions emanated from a group of sheds to the rear of Marconi's New Street Works.

The tests were broadcast on 2,750 metres. Some of the tests contained readings from Bradshaw's railway timetable; others featured gramophone records and recitals by local musicians. One such musician was Miss Winifred Sayer, a local soprano, who became the first woman broadcaster. She sang in the main transmission room amidst all the noisy equipment

Many radio amateurs and ship's radio operators tuned in to the transmissions. Reports were received from as far away as Belgium, Norway and Portugal. This greatly encouraged Marconi and on 15th June a 30-minute recital by Dame Nellie Melba was broadcast. Rather wisely they did not place her in the noisy transmission room. Instead Melba sang in a small shed well away from the equipment.

Before the broadcast Dame Nellie was shown around Marconi's factory. As part of her tour she was shown the huge 450 ft twin towers that would transmit her recital. Her guide explained to her that from the top of the mast her voice would be heard throughout the world. "Young Man", she retorted, "if you think I'm going to climb up there you are very much mistaken".

Dame Nellie's recital was sponsored by the Daily Mail and received a lot of coverage in the press. It was also heard all over Europe. Countless other transmissions of music were made throughout the summer.

Melba was not the only opera legend to sing at Chelmsford. Five weeks later the Danish Tenor Lauritz Melchior performed in the studio. He had to be placed well away from the microphone as his powerful voice could have upset the delicate equipment. Shortly afterwards the famous contralto Dame Clara Butt also made an appearance at New Street.

The first complete wireless receivers appeared in the UK in 1920. They were made by BTH – The British Thomson Houston Company. They were joined a year later by Burnham & Company and L. McMichael Limited. Receivers in those days were extremely unselective and speech and music required a fairly large space on the long wave band. Broadcasts continued until the autumn, when the Post Office stopped issuing the authorisation that was required for each transmission. This was because of complaints of interference with military communications.

In the USA commercial broadcasting was a great success. There was a large demand for receivers, and by 1922 numerous stations were broadcasting. This fuelled interest in Britain, and manufacturers fervently wanted to emulate the success of their American counterparts.

Eventually the Marconi Company was permitted to resume weekly test transmissions. This experimental station was based at Writtle, a small village two miles west of Chelmsford. 2MT was the first British radio station to make regular entertainment broadcasts. Transmissions began on 14 February 1922 from an ex-Army hut next to the Marconi laboratories. Initially the station only had 200 watts and transmitted on 700m (428 kHz) on Tuesdays from 2000 to 2030.

The first transmission was far from a success. The signal was weak and the sound was muffled. However things did gradually improve. These early tests consisted mainly of gramophone records but a live concert was broadcast on April 11th. Miss Nora Scott sang three songs accompanied by her pianist. Melchior also made his debut on 2MT a few weeks later.

'Two Emma Toc', in the phonetic alphabet of the day, was a surprising success. The station was fronted by the eccentric Captain Peter Pendleton Eckersley, a Marconi engineer. Eckersley, known as PPE by his friends, was no shrinking violet and his enthusiasm pervaded the whole proceedings. PPE liked to experiment with sound and would use whatever was lying around to make unusual noises. He would perform spontaneous comedy sketches and improvise operatic parodies. His regular announcement, "This is Two Emma Toc, Writtle testing, Writtle testing", delivered in his jocular style became extremely well known in a very short space of time.

The station even produced a piece of drama. The balcony scene from Cyrano was chosen as it's staged in semi-darkness with virtually stationary actors and so Eckersley considered it highly suitable for broadcasting. The main actress of the piece boasted the marvellous sobriquet of Uggy Travers

The Writtle transmission station suspended transmissions in January 1923. Peter Eckersley eventually became the first Chief Engineer of the BBC until 1929, when he was sacked by John Reith after divorcing his wife.

The Marconi Company was given another licence to operate a transmitter at Marconi House, in London. This was the famous '2LO', which started broadcasting on May 11th 1922. The Marconi employee in charge of 2LO's output was Arthur Burrows. His background was journalism but Burrows had helped train radio operators during the First World War. Burrows quickly realised that wireless telephony had great potential in the field of mass entertainment and journalism.

The initial broadcasts were speech only but permission was eventually granted to broadcast music. The first concert was transmitted on June 24th 1922 and included a cellist, a pianist and a baritone. The artistes performed in the cinema on the top floor of Marconi House.

Stanton Jeffries was appointed Musical Director and there followed a series of regular concerts culminating in four performances daily during the first 'All-British Wireless Exhibition and Convention'. This event took place in the Horticultural Hall in Westminster between the 30th September and the 7th October 1922. This exhibition provided many with their first encounter with radio. 2LO's output was relayed via a powerful valve set with large speakers placed around the hall.

Also in September, the station kept the listeners informed on progress during the 'King's Cup Air Race'. The Air Ministry provided daily reports. 2LO broadcast its first comedy programme on the 20th October. 'A Cockney Fragment from Life' was written and performed by Helena Millais as 'Our Lizzie'.

2LO's power was 1.5kW on a frequency of 840 kHz. Programmes were initially broadcast for just an hour each day. However 2LO was only allowed to transmit for seven minutes at a time. This was because the 'operator' had to listen on the wavelength for three minutes for possible instructions to close down. This restriction was finally lifted on January 8th 1923.

Marconi wasn't the only company interested in the new medium. In Manchester, the Metropolitan Vickers Company Limited commenced test broadcasts on May 16th 1922 from its own station identified as 2ZY. The broadcasts originated from the firm's base in Old Trafford.

Metropolitan Vickers concentrated mainly on heavy engineering but it did have a sister company called The Radio Communication Company. The RCC specialised in marine communication and they supplied most of the start up equipment.

The tests were organised by Kenneth Wright, an engineer in the Research Department of Metropolitan Vickers. Tests were sporadic at first and 2ZY didn't have a regular studio until July 1922. The transmitter was installed on October 25th and tests began in earnest shortly after. The regular tests relied heavily on gramophone records. A deal had been struck with the Gramophone Company to provide records free of charge. This was on the understanding that they would receive free publicity and no other company's records were used. The first live concert was broadcast on Halloween 1922 and used musical talent from within Metropolitan Vickers staff.

Birmingham would also get its own station. The Western Electric Company had played a large part in expanding the British telephone network. They had also developed a popular public address system.

The various technologies used by these systems meant that they were in a good position to enter the broadcasting field. However they had procrastinated more than Marconi and Metropolitan Vickers so they had to move fast if they were to be ready by the proposed start up date of November 1922.

Western Electric secured an agreement with the General Electric Company to house its station within their works at Witton in Birmingham. An engineer called A E Thompson was placed in charge of the operation. Thompson and his team managed to equip the studios and commence tests within three days.

The station utilised a new type of microphone used in Western Electric's public address system. The 'double button' carbon microphone increased the frequency response and was far superior to other types of microphones at the time. The transmitter was built in Western Electric's laboratories in London and transferred by steam lorry to the Birmingham site. The station was assigned the call sign 2WP.

2LO's engineers were anxious to check that 2WP wouldn't interfere with their broadcasts so the two broadcast simultaneously on the 5th November. No interference was subsequently reported.

Although the stations in London, Birmingham and Manchester were independent of each other they were unlikely to stay that way for long. The Post Office had come under severe pressure to allow national broadcasting and so they met with representatives from interested groups on May 18th 1922. At this point there had been 23 requests from applicants to start broadcasting. The Post Office asked them to come up with a mutual scheme for broadcasting. These discussions went on for five months without any proper proposal. At each meeting there was a large amount of conflict as each company vehemently protected its own interests.

The delay in reaching any agreement was criticised by the government and the press. Finally on October 18th a decision was made to form a single entity that would be responsible for broadcasting in Britain.

The British Broadcasting Committee was a transitory body, which lasted until the new company could be officially registered. This transitional period lasted until December and early broadcasts were announced as 'on behalf of the Broadcasting Committee'.

The efforts of the committee resulted in the formation of the British Broadcasting Company, which would establish a nationwide network of radio transmitters many of which had originally been owned by member companies, from which the BBC was to provide a national broadcasting service.

The British Broadcasting Company, Ltd. was incorporated under the 1908 to 1917 Companies Acts with a share capital of £100,000., with 99,993 cumulative ordinary shares valued at £1 each. The six largest companies provided the capital. These were Marconi, BTH, GEC, Western Electric, Metropolitan Vickers and the Radio Communication Company. Any British manufacturer or retailer could become a member by purchasing at least one £1 share.

This British Broadcasting Company would derive some income from a licence sold to listeners, the rest from the manufacture and sale of licenced receiving sets. Initially there weren't enough licences available so in many cases a personal letter was sent out giving permission to listen. These letters later enclosed a permit to be carried at all times.

In the early days there were different types of licences. The broadcast licence fee was introduced on November 1st 1922 and cost 10 shillings. This applied to listeners who purchased one of the official BBC sets. The constructor's licence was introduced in October 1923 at 15 shillings. This was for amateurs wishing to construct their own receivers using British-made components only. This licence was only available briefly and was terminated in July 1924. The 'Receiving Licence' was introduced in January 1925 and all previous forms of licences were abolished. These licences covered all wireless sets in your home but you were required to have a separate licence if you had a car radio.

Half the licence-fee went to the BBC and the rest to the six manufacturers mentioned previously. Receivers manufactured in the UK were required to carry a distinctive label indicating that royalties had been paid.

In addition the listeners had to pay two tariffs. The first was based upon the various components in the receiver and went to the BBC.

The second was a levy of 12s.6d per valve-holder, which would go to the Marconi Company as a royalty in return for allowing their patents to be used.

On Tuesday 14th November 1922, the BBC officially took control of 2LO and started broadcasting in the medium waveband. However it did so without a licence from the Post Office. The Licence was eventually issued retrospectively in January 1923. The broadcasts emanated from the seventh floor of Marconi House on the Strand. Initially the power was 100 watts on 350 metres (857 kHz).

The first programme was the evening news read by the Programme Director Arthur Burrows. He read each bulletin twice, once quickly and once slowly. Burrows then asked listeners to say what they preferred. The first bulletin included details of a speech given by the Conservative leader Bonar Law, the opening of the Old Bailey sessions, the aftermath of a 'rowdy meeting' involving Winston Churchill, a train robbery, the sale of a Shakespearean first folio, fog in London - and "the latest billiards scores". Due to pressure from the newspaper industry, the BBC was not allowed to transmit its news bulletins until after 7pm. This was so newspaper sales would not be lost to a BBC radio news service.

The first chairman of the British Broadcasting Company was Lord Gainford, a former Postmaster-General. The new organisation didn't have a General Manager at its helm during its inception. However the British Broadcasting Company eventually appointed John Reith as its first General Manager on December 14th 1922. Reith, a minister's son, had been born in Stonehaven in the North East of Scotland in 1889. His family moved to Glasgow while Reith was an infant. After his education at Glasgow Academy he served an engineering apprenticeship where he specialised in radio communication.

His strict Presbyterian upbringing had a big influence on his life and greatly affected his demeanour. The dour, humourless Scot described his early life when interviewed for John Freeman's 'Face to Face' programme in the 1950s. Reith portrayed a life of austerity and in his own words he 'never learned that life was for living'.

Although he was a difficult man to like he turned out to be the perfect man for the job. Reith knew nothing about broadcasting but relished the challenge his new position presented him. He immediately began innovating, experimenting and organising, Under his leadership the BBC was turned from what was a handful of experimental stations run by wireless manufacturers into a cohesive organisation with a mission to 'Educate, Inform and Entertain'. He directed staff to make quality broadcasts with a strong moral underpinning.

The other stations in Birmingham and Manchester also transferred operations to the BBC. The Birmingham station, now renamed 5IT, started broadcasting at 17:20 on November 15th. One hour and forty minutes later, 2ZY went on the air in Manchester.

The 15th November was polling day in the 1922 general election and all three stations stayed on air until 1am to carry results phoned through from Reuters. There had been prolonged dialogue regarding news. It was agreed that Reuters would supply a summary for use after 6pm. This was dictated over the telephone to Marconi House and passed again by telephone to the other stations.

Frederick Percy Edgar was the General Manager and opening announcer for 5IT. Edgar was a former music hall act who became a director of a concert agency in Birmingham. He was approached initially by the Western Electric Company to supply artists to perform on the radio station. He was surprised to receive an offer shortly afterwards to manage the station itself. His friends and colleagues advised him to turn the job down as radio would be just a passing craze but he accepted and became the BBC's senior Regional Director.

5IT pioneered many innovations, from employing the first full time announcers to launching children's programmes. 'Children's Hour' was the brainchild of A E Thompson who broadcast as 'Uncle Tom'. The practice of the children's announcers adopting the appellation of Aunt' or 'Uncle' was also adopted at other stations. Published stories were forbidden due to copyright so Thompson invented stories about a cat called Susan. These stories were based on a grotesque china cat he found in a junk shop. He was later joined by another engineer F H Amis who became 'The Fairy Dustman'.

Many music hall acts were given the opportunity to broadcast. Thompson recalled one act from the Aston Hippodrome who didn't fully grasp the concept of sound broadcasting. The woman flounced around the studio as if on stage with Thompson trailing behind her holding the microphone on a long lead. After this incident a small podium was built out of crates and the performers were told to stand on it and not move.

General Electric's premises at Witton were unsuitable for the BBC's long-term aims and alternative accommodation was sought. In August 1923 the Birmingham station moved to the second floor of a large building at 105 New Street. The new premises included a studio, control room and offices. There were also two other rooms set aside for a reception and band room. The transmitter was moved from Witton to a power station at Summer Lane.

2ZY in Manchester also moved to a more central location. The station relocated to the fifth floor of a warehouse in Dickinson Street during the summer of 1923. The new premises were adjacent to the Manchester Corporation Power Station where the aerial mast was erected. The close proximity of studio, transmitter and aerial mast negated the need for any GPO landline. The move to Dickinson Street coincided with Kenneth Wright's departure for a senior post in London and a replacement station manager was sought.

2ZY's new station manager, Dan Godfrey Junior, created an orchestra of twelve players known as the 2ZY Orchestra. He also initiated an opera company and there began a regular series of live music broadcasts. Many works, principally by British composers, were given their first broadcast performances by the 2ZY Orchestra. These included Holst's 'The Planets', Elgar's 'Enigma Variations' and 'The Dream of Gerontius'. The 2ZY Orchestra was eventually renamed the Northern Wireless Orchestra in 1926.

5NO, the Newcastle station, started broadcasting in December 1922. The BBC moved into brand new premises in the city centre. The annual rent for 24 Eldon Square was £250 p.a. This was the first time that a BBC station had not benefited from existing studios used by previous test stations.

The transmitter site was located a mile away from 5NO's studios at the stable yards of the Co-operative Wholesale Society in West Blandford Street. The BBC had rented one of the stables to house the transmitter and a nearby factory chimney supported the aerial.

The first day of broadcasting was set to be December 23rd 1922. At the last moment, technical problems arose when trying to connect the transmitter to the studio. Therefore the cast and crew of the opening broadcast were forced to broadcast from the stable yard instead. The engineers wheeled empty carts into the yard and placed chairs on them and microphones were connected to the nearby transmitter. Tom Payne, the Station Director, made the opening announcement and played his violin. There followed several songs from May Osborne and a cello recital from a Mr Griffiths.

The studio link was ready the following day and this is officially considered to be the opening date of 5NO. There was a slight problem during the first broadcast from the studios when a howling dog, kennelled nearby, could be heard faintly in the background.

Tom Payne's tenure as Station Director was brief and Bertram Fryer replaced him in March 1923. Fryer adopted the best features of other stations. As 'Uncle Jack' he initiated the Fairy Flower League and encouraged youngsters to develop an interest in animals and plants. Fryer also set up receivers with loudspeakers in local cinemas so patrons could listen to 5NO while watching a silent film.

The first BBC outside broadcast took place on January 8th 1923. Post Office engineers installed a quarter mile long lead-sheathed cable between the Covent Garden Opera House and Marconi House. Mozart's 'Magic Flute' was transmitted to an extremely appreciative audience. Announcer Stanton Jeffries was placed in the prompter's box to convey what was happening during silent periods on stage. The operas 'Hansel and Gretel', 'Pagliacci' and 'Siegfried' were all transmitted on subsequent evenings. The season climaxed on January 17th with a performance of La Bohème starring Dame Nellie Melba. Harrods remained open that night so customers could listen to the event in the Georgian Restaurant.

The first experimental transatlantic radio relay took place in the early hours of November 26th 1923. The BBC used eight stations throughout Britain for the tests, all relaying the same programme from London. For the first fifteen minutes nothing was heard. Then faint, unintelligible speech was heard. A telegram was sent to the BBC asking for a piano solo. Three minutes later the notes of a piano were heard, followed by the words "Hello America". A month later, on the 30th December, the first continental broadcast to the UK was made by landline from Radiola in Paris.

The BBC's station in London continued to innovate. The first religious address on the BBC was broadcast on Christmas Eve

1922. The Reverend John Mayo, the Rector of St Mary's Whitechapel, broadcast two sermons that day. The first one was broadcast during a programme for children and he returned later in the evening to speak to the adults.

In April 1924 the BBC decided to broadcast a regular religious service and chose St Martin-in-the-Fields church as the venue. This soon became a regular monthly feature, with Dick Sheppard, 'the radio parson', sharing his pulpit with other clergy.

Certain sectors of the entertainment industry felt threatened by radio. The Theatrical Manager's Association withdrew its support, as it feared the new medium would affect ticket sales. Other impresarios agreed and prevented their artists from participating in broadcasts. The embargo stayed in place throughout the BBC's early years.

The Newspaper Association also viewed the BBC with suspicion. During the spring of 1923, John Reith received an ultimatum from the Newspaper Publishers' Association warning him that if the corporation didn't pay a hefty fee, none of the association's publications would carry radio listings. Although the embargo was short-lived, it gave Reith the idea of publishing a dedicated listings magazine. And so the first edition of The Radio Times, 'the official organ of the BBC', duly appeared on September 28th 1923.

Radio Times was a joint venture between the BBC and publisher George Newnes Ltd, who produced, printed and distributed the magazine. The Radio Times quickly established a good reputation. It used the leading writers and illustrators of the day and the covers from the special editions of this period are now regarded as design classics. Weekly sales had reached 750,000 by the end of 1924 and the BBC assumed full editorial control in 1925. By 1937 the magazine was printed and published in-house, where it has remained ever since.

The Radio Times was a late addition to the newsagents' stands. There were four magazines dedicated to radio on sale as early as December 1922. These were Amateur Wireless, Popular Wireless Weekly, The Broadcaster and Wireless World.

2LO's initial broadcasts were estimated to have reached an audience of about 18,000. The BBC's home was still Marconi's headquarters in the Strand. However it was decided to seek suitable accommodation of its own. It settled on the Institution of Electrical Engineers' building in Savoy Hill, near the Embankment. The premises were opened on 1st May 1923. The first studio was built on the third floor and by 1926 there were five studios in use.

The atmosphere at Savoy Hill was friendly, but idiosyncratic. Each evening a rat-catcher looked for vermin and office boys in rubber gloves puffed germicide everywhere to prevent coughs and sneezes among the broadcasters.

The engineers were keen to avoid the acoustic problems that dogged transmissions from Marconi House. Each studio floor had a thick wall to wall carpet and the walls were lined with five layers of canvas. Each layer was stretched on a wooden frame and placed an inch apart. A sixth layer of yellow net curtains completed the acoustic barrier.

Taking centre stage in the Savoy Hill studios was a brand new microphone. The 'Magnetophone' or 'Marconi Round Sykes', weighed 25-pounds and was trundled round on a wheeled base. The microphone was enclosed in a wire mesh and was likened by the engineers to 'a meat safe on a large tea trolley'. The contraption was almost 5ft tall and required a row of car batteries to power it.

Henry Joseph Round, Marconi's Chief Engineer, designed the new microphone. Round had joined the Marconi Company in 1902 shortly after Marconi made his transatlantic wireless transmission. He was sent to the USA where he experimented with a variety of different aspects of radio technology.

The First World War broke out in 1914 and Round was seconded to Military Intelligence with the rank of Captain. He set up a chain of direction finding stations along the Western Front. These stations proved so successful that another set was installed in England. For his services during the war, Round was awarded the Military Cross. When war broke out again in 1939, the British Government again called on his services. This time he was involved in developing Sonar.

The inaugural broadcast from Savoy Hill featured speeches by Lord Birkenhead, Sir William Bull and Lord Gainford. Lord Birkenhead caused some concern by failing to appear at the appointed time. Enquiries revealed he was dining next door at the Savoy Hotel and a deputation was hastily despatched to get him. When he finally appeared he seemed 'unsteady on his feet' but delivered his speech perfectly.

The Band of the Grenadier Guards provided the music and entertainer Norman Long was on hand to provide light relief. Norman Long was the first entertainer to be 'made' by radio. He made his debut on the BBC on November 28th 1922. Long's music hall slogan 'A Song, a Smile and a Piano' was changed to 'A Song, a Joke and a Piano' on the basis that you can't *hear* a smile.

By May 1924, every available space in the Institute of Electrical Engineers building was utilised so they expanded into the adjacent Savoy Hill Mansions, part of which had been destroyed in a Zeppelin raid in 1917.

The BBC continued to expand. The first new station to start broadcasting in 1923 was 5WA Cardiff, which commenced transmissions on February 13th. It proved difficult to find suitable premises and compromises had to be made. The only location that could be found was cramped rooms situated above a cinema across from Cardiff Castle.

The studio location made soundproofing difficult and the noise of trams trundling by on the street below was a permanent backdrop to broadcasts. The transmitters were located a mile away at an electricity sub-station in Ninian Park Road. Rex Palmer was the Station Director but his tenure at Cardiff was brief as he was appointed to a similar role at 2LO in April.

A month later, on March 6th 1923, Glasgow got its regional station when 5SC started transmissions. The great and the good were in attendance at its inaugural broadcast. The sound of bagpipes was followed by the BBC's General Manager John Reith's opening announcement. Reith then introduced BBC Chairman Lord Gainford, The Principal of Glasgow University and Glasgow's Lord Provost, who all made short speeches.

Early employees at 5SC included M. M. Dewar, A. H. A. Paterson and Kathleen Garscadden. These three performed administrative duties in addition to on air duties. They were regulars on Children's Hour and were known as Uncle Mungo, Uncle Alex and Auntie Cyclone respectively. The Station Director was H. A. Carruthers, who took his position shortly after the inaugural broadcast. Carrutthers was a well-respected musician and conductor.

Glasgow's headquarters consisted of several cramped rooms in an attic at Rex House, 202 Bath Street. It may have lacked space but 5SC enjoyed the latest technology. The studio boasted a Western Electric double button carbon microphone and amplifier. The Marconi Q transmitter was situated at the Port Dundas Power Station. The aerial was slung between two chimneys, which towered above the complex.

The citizens of the North East of Scotland joined the radio age on a cold blustery evening on October 10th 1923. The Aberdeen radio station was assigned the call sign '2BD' and began broadcasting on 495 metres. At 6.50p.m. the sound of pipe music was heard, followed by station announcements read by Station Director R. E Jeffery. He had been the principal actor in many important touring companies before running the Aldwych Theatre in London.

The BBC rented accommodation at the rear of Aberdeen Electrical Engineering's property at 17 Belmont Street. Access to the premises was gained by the narrow stairway at the rear of the shop. On the second floor were a couple of small offices and a large room. The room was an old meeting hall, which overlooked the main Aberdeen to Inverness railway line. The area was converted in to a rudimentary studio by draping heavy black curtains on the wall to deaden the noise from the passing trains. The studio was particularly affected by the vagaries of the North East Scotland weather. No central heating or air conditioning meant the temperature veered between freezing cold in the winter to boiling hot during the summer.

The Marquis of Aberdeen performed the official opening ceremony at 9.00pm followed by music from the Military Band of the 2nd Gordon Highlanders. There were several aural delights for the listener during that inaugural transmission. A contralto, Miss May Lymburn, performed several light operatic numbers throughout the evening and entertainer Robert Murray performed several selections from his repertoire at the piano.

The transmitter was located in the premises of the Aberdeen Steam Laundry Company in Claremont Street. Perhaps this was taking the idea of Steam Radio too literally. From there the signal was sent to the aerial, which was strung up between two tall Marconi masts. It was perhaps unwise to site the studios near to several electrical generators as these often interfered with the signal. Despite the low power, the initial broadcasts were heard in Norway and 2BD's output was clearly picked up in the United States during International Radio Week in November 1924.

Bournemouth (6BM) opened seven days after the Aberdeen station on October 17th 1923. The purpose-built studio premises were located at Holdenhurst Road. The transmitter was situated 1.5 miles way at North Cemetery, Bushey Road. Bertram Fryer moved from Newcastle to become the Station Director.

Each station was responsible for its own output, provided they adhered to the guidelines issued from London. To help fill the broadcast hours, the London office would often send up a large leather trunk filled with sheet music and material for the local actors and musicians to perform. A team of peripatetic performers also travelled around the regions doing one-night stands at each location. Their gruelling fortnightly schedule would take them to stations throughout Scotland, Northern Ireland, Wales and England.

To give a flavour of the type of output these early stations provided, let's look at some of the programmes that 2BD in Aberdeen transmitted.

Technical limitations meant certain types of programmes were more prevalent. The single person talk was a necessary requirement of the early days in broadcasting because there was only one microphone in the studio. The microphone was the 'Marconi Round Sykes' type enclosed in a wire mesh. This gauze structure gave the technical boffins loads of headaches, especially in summer. Bluebottles frequently got inside from the bottom of the stand and became trapped in the mesh. When this happened, all the listener would hear was a loud humming noise and the broadcast would have to be suspended while the offending insect was removed.

Station 2BD became one of the first stations to broadcast a weekly 15-minute sports programme. Peter Craigmile, the international football referee, would preview the week's forthcoming events. The Aberdeen Station was also responsible for another broadcasting first when it transmitted a Gaelic language programme in 1923.

Programmes normally began at 3.30pm with closedown happening between 10.30pm and midnight. Each broadcast day lasted for seven hours and, as there was no opt out facility, consisted entirely of live broadcasts. Charity events, community singing and special weather forecasts for farmers were frequently heard. Light music and comedy shows were particularly well received.

Local performers and musicians were enlisted to help and the Aberdeen station could act as a springboard to greater things. Local harmonica player Donald Davidson secured a recording contract with Beltona Records after being discovered on 2BD.

The 2BD Repertory Company was established to perform adaptations of the classics as well as numerous offerings in the local vernacular. These were mostly one-act plays with a handful of characters. For example on Thursday 1st August 1926 the listeners were treated to a Scots comedy by Jessie R.F. Allan called 'The Dark Gentleman'.

One popular drama series was centred on a fictitious castle in Aberdeenshire. 'The House at Rosieburn' told the tale of a witch burnt at the stake who, before she died, placed a curse on the inhabitants. One actor, playing a witch finder in the series, was the envy of his colleagues when he was given an official sanction to utter the line "Come on you old bitch!" Although quite tame by today's standards this was considered quite outrageous language at the time.

The station had its own 12-piece orchestra, formed in 1924, to provide musical entertainment. These interludes would prove to be extremely popular with the listening public.

In accordance with BBC policy, the musicians would dress in full evening wear for every performance. The only time they were permitted to remove their jackets was on particularly hot days during the summer. There was no air conditioning in those days and they couldn't open a window because of the noise of the nearby railway. The performers had no choice but to sweat it out.

Their double bass player once unwittingly put the station off the air during a heat wave. Perspiring profusely he looked down and noticed a plug in a nearby wall socket. In a fit of pique he bent down and unplugged what he thought was the radiator. Unfortunately it turned out to be the socket for the one and only microphone and it was several minutes before the error was realised. The orchestra was reduced to an octet in December 1926 before eventually being disbanded in October 1929.

In addition, popular music hall artistes were invited to perform when they were in the area. Mabel Constanduros was a character actress who was incredibly popular in the early days of wireless. She performed comedy monologues as various members of the Buggins family. Mabel appeared before the 2BD microphone on February 3rd 1928 in a programme with the catchy title 'Mrs Buggins gives a party in the Aberdeen Studio'.

Each station provided special programmes for children and Aberdeen was no exception. Each week a number of eager youngsters were invited along to the Belmont Street Studios to hear a story from Winifred Manners or 'Auntie Win' as she was known. These children's broadcasts became extremely popular and youngsters were clamouring to pay their shilling to join the junior listener's club. They received an enamel badge and a different coloured membership card each year. By 1928 the Radio Circle boasted 19,000 members nationwide.

The establishment of 6BM in Bournemouth fulfilled the initial obligation to build eight stations in the main areas of population. However the BBC needed to cover the widest population in the quickest way possible in order to make the service profitable for the company's shareholders. The obvious solution was to keep adding to the initial stations. However the existing high-power stations could not increase their power without causing mutual interference.

The Covent Garden Opera broadcasts had proved it was possible to use a post office land line over short distances. Therefore the BBC wondered if it would be possible to relay a programme from one part of the country to another. They decided to experiment and hire two lines from Birmingham to London. They used one for communication between the studios and the other to convey the broadcast itself. On March 20th 1923 a musical programme was relayed from Birmingham to London. The experiment was repeated on the 16th April, only this time from Glasgow. The engineers were pleased with the quality even though there was some distortion on high notes.

The signal needed to be boosted so that the simultaneous broadcast would reach outlying transmitters. In order to do this a series of amplifiers would be used in each location. Two further tests were carried out using this method but these were less satisfactory as severe interference was heard. Eventually the problems were ironed out and the era of simultaneous broadcasting had arrived.

The new technique also enabled the news to be broadcast directly from London. This ended the frustrating nightly practice of phoning all the provincial stations and dictating the news script to them. The first simultaneous news broadcast was read by John Reith on August 29th 1923.

Simultaneous broadcasting was seen as a way to broadcast special programmes to a wider audience. It caught on quickly and by the end of 1923 nearly a third of 2LO's output was being relayed to the provincial stations. This figure had risen to 50% by the time 1924 had concluded.

When new stations were introduced they were classed as either a 'main' or 'relay' station. The relay stations would receive programmes from the nearest main city studio via telephone circuits. However each station had a studio to opt out of the main transmissions if required. The first relay station was Sheffield (2FL) which first transmitted on November 16th 1923. The Sheffield station was located in the Union Grinding Wheel Company premises in Corporation Street.

Several other stations joined the list in 1924. There was 5PY in Plymouth, which first broadcast on the 26th March. The studio complex was located at Athenaeum Lane and the 100-watt transmitter was situated at the sugar refinery in Mill Street.

2EH in Edinburgh started relaying 5SC on May Day 1924. The Edinburgh office was located in the back premises of a music shop at 79 George Street. 2EH broadcast every afternoon and also on Friday nights.

Relays of 2ZY were introduced during the summer. These covered Liverpool, Leeds, Bradford, Nottingham, Hull and Stoke on Trent. 2BE in Belfast joined the list on the 15th September. 2DE started to relay the Aberdeen programmes to Dundee from premises in Lochee Road on November 9th 1924.

Finally 5SX relayed 5WA's programmes to Swansea, commencing on December 12th 1924, from the top floor of the Oxford Buildings on Union Street. Alderman John Lewis, Mayor of Swansea, was in attendance as Wilfrid Goatman made the opening announcement.

The British Broadcasting Company Ltd did not sell air time for commercials. Its licence did allow for it to carry sponsored programming and eight such sponsored broadcasts were aired in 1925. However its main income was still derived by the sale of radio sets and the licence fee. By the autumn of 1924, the GPO had issued over 1 million receiving licences. The BBC had 20 radio transmitting stations in operation and 465 employees.

The original stations reached about half of the population, with signals that were strong enough to be received by a crystal set. The 'listeners in' as they were called, had to show a remarkable dedication to listen to these early broadcasts. In the 1920s buying a radio was a very expensive proposition and only the rich would have been able to buy a commercially built radio.

The alternative to buying a commercially made set was to build a home-made radio. The simplest receiver was a crystal set, which used a mineral crystal as a rectifier, and enabled the listener to tune in the station on headphones. This was assuming they were within range of a station and could locate a receptive part of the crystal using a wire probe called a 'cat's whisker'.

A crystal set had no power from mains or batteries, and relied on the energy from the radio waves that were collected in its large long-wire aerial to work. The aerial for a crystal set would have to have been many tens of yards long for anything to be heard.

To obtain greater range or volume, a valve receiver was needed. This would amplify the radio signals and the sounds so that weaker signals would be heard. A valve radio would require more electronic components and both low voltage and high voltage batteries for it to work, making it a more expensive proposition. A valve cost a week's wages and was extremely fragile and easily damaged. The early valves also had a relatively short life and so needed frequent replacement.

A large high-tension battery and a low-tension accumulator provided the power. They could be recharged like a modern mobile phone or laptop battery. The difference was, these beasts weighed several pounds and were full of corrosive acid so a slow careful walk to the local dealer was a necessity. Most radio owners had two, one to use and one being charged. You could easily spot a wireless enthusiast in those days by the acid burns on his hands. Wireless dealers, as well as cycle shops and garages, would recharge batteries and accumulators for about 6d.

One person could listen on headphones, but a loudspeaker was needed for a family to 'listen in'. These were usually metal or wooden horns fixed to a telephone receiver. These horn speakers were eventually replaced by the moving coil type, which appeared just before 1930. This is the type we still use today.

The early valve receivers were mostly of the tuned radio frequency type, which often had a confusing array of different switches and knobs on the front panel. Tuning in a station required the operation of numerous controls, and to change waveband sometimes required the insertion of different tuning coils. Many receivers had a reaction control that adjusted the sensitivity and selectivity of the receiver. The receiver would oscillate and act like a transmitter if the reaction control was adjusted too far, consequently interfering with everyone else's receiver in the neighbourhood.

The modern type of receiver appeared in 1925. The super heterodyne, or superhet for short, was a highly sensitive and selective receiver, with a vastly reduced selection of tuning controls. In those days mains electricity was provided by hundreds of small companies, which supplied electricity in a variety of different voltages, frequencies and even D.C. The national grid was set up in the early 1930s and standardised the supply. This made it much easier to produce mains power supplies for receivers. It also helped to establish mains powered radios. Mains powered receivers and battery eliminators first appeared in 1926. The first mains powered receiver to entirely dispense with batteries was the 'Baby Grand', made by Gambrell Brothers Limited.

One of the more unusual manufacturers of radio products was Meccano Ltd. The company manufactured a model construction system enabling purchasers to build working models and mechanical devices. A kit comprised re-usable metal strips, plates, angle girders, wheels, axles and gears, with nuts and bolts to connect the pieces.

The radio kit contained Meccano parts, a telephone earpiece, a crystal, and 'one or two inexpensive fittings'. However when the kit was first advertised, the construction of radio receivers was not permitted without first obtaining a constructors licence. Therefore a fully assembled set was introduced so that by December 1923 the Meccano Magazine carried an advertisement for two Crystal Receivers. The same magazine also contained an article by John Reith, the BBC's recently appointed General Manager, voicing his approval.

The new radio technology was advancing so quickly that other companies rapidly overtook Meccano. It's hard to establish how many sets might have been sold. By October 1925 Meccano were advertising just one receiver. In April 1928 the Meccano Magazine announced a 'Grand New Meccano Model-building competition'. The prizes included thirteen Meccano Radio Crystal Receiving Sets and thirty single telephone receivers. In May 1928 the competition prizes included Meccano Double Headphones. These competitions were probably a good way of disposing of the remaining stock.

During this period many people could not afford to buy a radio for the home. However there was an affordable alternative available to potential listeners in major towns and cities. For a weekly fee, usually a shilling, subscribers to wired relay networks received the BBC services without the need for a wireless set.

The first service of this kind appeared in 1928 and proliferated over the next three decades. The companies who provided these systems usually had a mast with the necessary equipment to receive the radio signals off the air. These masts were often at an elevated site that afforded good reception. The signals were then diffused via a cable network to homes in the area. At its height, radio relay services were used in over one million homes throughout the country.

Subscribers simply had a loudspeaker that could be switched on and off and a dial that could select one of the three BBC radio programme services. The loudspeaker required no battery or mains power, and in many households it would often be left on all day long.

The BBC broadcast the chimes of Big Ben for the first time in December 1923. A couple of months later, another time related tradition was introduced. The Greenwich Time Signal was first broadcast in February 1924. The 'pips' as they're more generally known were the brainchild of Frank Dyson, ninth Astronomer Royal. The six-pip time signal was devised in discussion with Frank Hope-Jones, inventor of the free pendulum clock, who had originally advocated a five-pip signal. The sixth pip signals the start of the next minute.

The pips were originally controlled by two mechanical clocks located in the Royal Greenwich Observatory that had electrical contacts attached to their pendula. Two clocks were used in case of a breakdown. The clocks sent a signal each second to the BBC which was then converted to the audible oscillatory tone used in the broadcast. Before the BBC started using the pips, a pianist in a studio would play the tune of the Westminster chimes, synchronising the 'bong' with the clock in the studio.

On January 15th 1924, the BBC broadcast its first specially commissioned 'listening play' as it was dubbed. 'A Comedy of Danger' by Richard Hughes was about a group of people trapped in a Welsh coal mine. To help with atmosphere the listener was encouraged to turn out the lights and listen in the dark. The producers encountered several problems when it came to sound effects. The acoustics of the studio could not recreate a vast cavernous mineshaft so the actors (Joyce Kennedy, Kenneth Kent, and H. R. Hignett) had to place their heads in buckets.

A male voice choir were enlisted as the script called for 'distant snatches of hymn-singing'. However the men were very enthusiastic and once started nothing could stop them. The producer put them in the corridor outside with a soundproof door he could open and shut when required.

An explosion proved to be trickier as any large noise would have disturbed the transmitting equipment and put the BBC off the air. Therefore instead of a loud bang, the listeners heard a muffled thud. This was not what a group of invited journalists heard. The gentlemen of the press were ushered into a private room to listen to the play and so at the appropriate point an engineer concocted a substitute explosion in the room next door. The 'explosion' gained enthusiastic approval from the press. They never discovered they had heard it through the wall.

Another 'first' happened on April 23rd 1924 when the first broadcast by a reigning monarch was transmitted. Millions heard King George V open the Wembley Empire exhibition. Traffic was stopped on Oxford Street as crowds gathered to listen on loud speakers.

The Theatrical Manager's Association's embargo was eventually lifted and many music hall acts auditioned for the BBC. Not every act was suited to the new medium and many found it hard to perform in an empty room with no interaction from the audience. Many famous music hall acts failed to make the transition.

Those acts that could adapt found that it boosted their careers enormously. Willie Rouse, who came to be known as 'Wireless Willie', was extremely adept at improvising. His spontaneous gags were usually at the expense of the announcer or accompanist. Rouse was immensely popular but his radio career was short-lived. Wireless Willie died in 1928 at the age of 51.

John Henry had failed to make it big in the theatre but he found his niche in broadcasting. Henry specialised in monologues delivered in a droll Yorkshire accent. His idiosyncratic tales usually featured his wife 'Blossom and his dog 'Erbert'.

Some of the early stars of radio were rather unusual in that they didn't come from a show business background. Sir Walford Davies introduced the first schools broadcast in 1924 and embarked on a series of regular talks on music. His talks were knowledgeable but never opinionated and Davies had a sense of intimacy that remains the key to successful broadcasting

Sir Oliver Lodge had already occupied a key position in the history of radio. Lodge was well known in radio history as the inventor of the 'tuned circuit' but his ability to explain difficult scientific subjects clearly and simply endeared him to the audience. He was totally relaxed in front of a microphone and would often pause while searching for the correct word or phrase. After being introduced Lodge would clear his throat and proceed with his talk. This throaty growl became his 'signature tune'.

A J Allen was another regular contributor of talks who seemed to be making it up as he went along. However his pauses were cleverly contrived to give the impression of spontaneity. In reality all his talks were well rehearsed and nothing was left to chance. It later emerged that A J Allen was the pseudonym of Leslie Lambert who held a top-secret post in the Government.

In 1925 the London masts were moved to a new more powerful transmitter at Selfridge's Department Store in Oxford Street. The transmitter was housed in a large hut on the roof and the aerial was supported on two 125ft pylons. The transmitter and masts remained at this site until 1929.

Early in 1926, a talk by Father Ronald Knox caused some controversy. 'Broadcasting from the Barricades' featured fictitious reports of rioting in London by the unemployed. Many listeners panicked and thought that Britain was in the throes of revolution.

The longest running programme in the history of British radio made its first appearance at this time. The Week's Good Cause was first broadcast on 24th January 1926.

The BBC was still in its infancy when the values laid down by John Reith were first put to the test. The organisation clashed with the government over editorial independence during the general strike. In May 1926, Britain's miners went on strike and in a move of solidarity other industry workers joined them. For nine days the nation's industry was at a standstill. At such a politically sensitive time the company had to tread carefully.

Radio was the only widely available source of news, as many of the newspapers were not published. There were barely any means of communication between authorities and the general public. The Conservative government published its own 'British Gazette'. This was launched and edited by the then Chancellor, Winston Churchill. However Churchill could see that radio was a more direct and adaptable medium and he lobbied Prime Minister Stanley Baldwin to commandeer the company.

John Reith argued that such a move would destroy the company's reputation for independence and impartiality. He put forward a persuasive defence and Baldwin ruled that the BBC should remain independent. This judgement did not please Churchill who complained bitterly about the decision. He later said, "It was monstrous not to use such an instrument to the best possible advantage".

Reith argued later that the Conservative, Labour and trade union perspectives had all been reported impartially. However the TUC and the Labour Party, led by Ramsay MacDonald, disagreed. They said the BBC refused airtime to their representatives. The BBC's reporting of the strike was guarded and far from comprehensive but historians now view it as reasonably fair.

The general strike happened when the BBC was in a period of transition. On March 5th 1926, a Parliamentary Committee lead by Lord Crawford published its broadcasting report. The committee recommended that broadcasting should be conducted by a public corporation 'acting as trustee for the national interest. It called for the termination of the British Broadcasting Company and the creation of a Crown chartered, non-commercial organisation.

The Crawford Committee also approved the general tone of John Reith's programming approach. Not surprisingly, he became the first Director General of the BBC when the company assets were dissolved and it became the British Broadcasting Corporation on the 1st January 1927.

BBC STATIONS – JANUARY 1927

Location	Station Type	Call Sign	Start Date	Wavelength (KHZ)	Wavelength (Metres)
Aberdeen	Main	2BD	10th October 1923	600	500
Belfast	Main	2BE	15th September 1924	980	306
Birmingham	Main	5IT	15th November 1922	610	492
Bournemouth	Main	6BM	17th October 1923	920	326
Bradford	Relay	2LS	8th July 1924	1180	254
Cardiff	Main	5WA	13th February 1923	850	353
Daventry	High	5XX	25th July 1925	187.5	1600
Dundee	Relay	2DE	9th November 1924	1040	288
Edinburgh	Relay	2EH	1st May 1924	1020	294
Glasgow	Main	5SC	6th March 1923	740	405
Hull	Relay	6KH	15th August 1924	1040	288
Leeds	Relay	2LS	8th July 1924	1080	278
Liverpool	Relay	6LV	11th June 1924	1010	297
London	Main	2LO	14th November 1922	830	361
Manchester	Main	2ZY	15th November 1922	780	385
Newcastle	Main	5NO	24th December 1922	960	312
Nottingham	Relay	5NG	16th September 1924	1090	275
Plymouth	Relay	5PY	28th March 1924	750	400
Sheffield	Relay	6FL	16th November 1923	1100	273
Stoke on Trent	Relay	6ST	21st October 1924	1040	288
Swansea	Relay	5SX	12th December 1924	1040	288

4

The British Broadcasting Corporation

On December 20th 1926, the Crown charter and licence agreements creating the new Crown chartered, non-commercial organisation were published. On December 31st 1926, the contracts of 773 British Broadcasting Company Ltd staff were terminated and, with the dissolution of the company, shareholders were paid at par value. The company assets were transferred to the British Broadcasting Corporation.

While the BBC was no longer an independent commercial company, the aim of the charter was that it would stay free of central government intervention and an appointed Board of Governors would oversee the corporation.

John Reith was honoured with a knighthood in December 1926. Under his leadership the BBC continued its mission to 'inform, educate and entertain'.

The General Post Office had issued 2¼ million receiving licences by 1927 and the new corporation had 21 stations broadcasting around the UK. Nearly all of the country could obtain at least one of these, even with low quality receivers. 85% of the population could receive a choice of programmes.

1927 saw a number of 'firsts'. The first live sport broadcast was transmitted on the 15th January. Teddy Wakelam commentated on the rugby union international between England and Wales. A week later the first football match was broadcast.

Christopher Stone presented a record programme on July 7th 1927 and became the first British disc-jockey. His relaxed, conversational style was at odds with the BBC's usual starchy form of presentation. Stone's programmes became highly popular and they lasted until 1934. He was barred from the BBC as a consequence of signing up for a show on Radio Luxembourg. Stone's fee for this show was £5,000, a princely sum at the time.

The BBC coat of arms was adopted in March 1927 to represent the purpose and values of the corporation. The crest of the coat of arms has a lion above the helmet which is the national animal of the UK. The lion indicates the BBC's British identity. The lion grasps a thunderbolt in its outstretched paw to represent broadcasting itself.

Below the lion is a shield. The globe in the shield signifies the wide range of the BBC's operations. Around the globe are seven estoiles, heraldic symbols for divine goodness and nobility. Their place in the shield enhances the representation of the scope and breadth of the corporation. They also symbolize the planets, other than the Earth, known at the time of the BBC's founding.

In heraldic language the two eagles which grasp the shield are 'supporters'. Eagles represent the natural pace of broadcasting. Both eagles have bugles suspended from their collars, representing the public service element of broadcasting. The coat of arms features the BBC motto, 'Nation shall speak peace unto Nation'. The motto is most likely based on biblical verses from the Book of Micah and the Book of Isaiah: 'Nation shall not lift up sword against nation; neither shall they learn war anymore'.

The BBC upheld its mandate 'to inform, educate and entertain' when it assumed responsibility of the Promenade Concerts in 1927. This British tradition had been held at Queen's Hall in London since 1895. The aim of the 'Proms' was to promote classical music to a wider audience. It did this by adopting a less formal approach and offering reduced ticket prices. However the enterprise was encountering financial difficulties until the BBC stepped in.

Some believed that broadcasting the concerts would reduce audience numbers but this fear proved groundless. The BBC continues to broadcast the Proms to this day. For the first three years the concerts were given by 'Sir Henry Wood and his Symphony Orchestra', until the BBC Symphony Orchestra was formed in 1930.

Another BBC magazine 'The Listener' made its first appearance on January 16th 1929. Its published aim was to be "a medium for intelligent reception of broadcast programmes by way of amplification and explanation of those features which cannot now be dealt with in the editorial columns of the Radio Times". It previewed major literary and musical broadcasts and reproduced written versions of broadcast talks. It also reviewed new books, and printed a selected list of the more intellectual broadcasts for the coming week.

Despite their popularity, the days of the local stations were numbered. It was no longer feasible for twenty BBC stations to continue on twenty different wavelengths. The initial network was proving wasteful and resources were being squandered by duplicating the same kind of programmes on each of the different stations.

In June 1924, A Long Wave transmitter was opened in Chelmsford that was intended to spread the wings of the BBC onto foreign shores. BBC management quickly realised that a sustained service could be supplied to most of Britain.

The experimental long wave station was deemed a great success and so a permanent site was sought. On July 25th 1925 the Long Wave transmitter was moved to a more centralised location at Daventry in Northamptonshire. The new powerful 25kW transmitter on 1562 metres (187.5 kHz) enabled improved coverage across the UK.

The problem of interference from abroad was also becoming serious. In America the random proliferation of stations had proved unworkable. In March 1925, an international conference was convened to prevent 'a chaos of the ether'. The conference was to regulate the frequencies and power used by each European country and the Geneva plan was eventually implemented in November 1926. However the agreement halved the number of medium wavelengths used by the BBC at that time.

The development of Post Office landlines between studios meant that a sustaining service from London could be provided to the outlying stations. The need and the impetus to make 100% local programmes faded.

Simultaneous broadcasting made it possible for the development of both the National Programme and the Regional Programmes. On August 21st 1927, the BBC opened a high power medium wave transmitter at Daventry. 5GB replaced the existing local stations in the English Midlands. The new transmitter required a power of between 30 and 50 kilowatts, bigger than any transmitter previously built.

That allowed the BBC National Programme to provide a service programmed from London for the majority of the population. The new service was broadcast from the former experimental long wave transmitter 5XX. This arrangement marked the start of a new policy - 'The Regional Scheme'. By combining the resources of the local stations into one regional station in each area, with a basic sustaining service from London, the BBC hoped to increase programme quality whilst also centralising the management of the radio service.

5GB was deemed to be a great success and there followed the establishment of seven regional services across the UK, each broadcasting programmes from its own local studio - The regions covered were Midlands, West, North, South East, Scottish, Welsh and N Ireland. Some local studios were retained to provide for programming from particular areas within each region.

With the development of both the National Programme and the Regional Programmes, the smaller local stations slowly died out - and with them went the experimental phase of broadcasting. These changes were also accompanied by changes in terminology. Transmitters were no longer referred to as stations and studios were to be called offices.

This new Regional Scheme required the BBC to build new, more powerful, transmitting stations that could carry both the National Programme and the Regional Programme services to the whole country. The first of these 'Twin Wave' stations to be built specifically for the Regional Scheme was Brookman's Park in Hertfordshire. This site was capable of providing signals to London and the South East. The station was a huge enterprise, using four large lattice towers; two towers were used to support the aerial system for each service.

The Brookman's Park station opened in 1929 using wavelengths of 261 metres for the National Programme at 70 kilowatts and 356 metres for the Regional Programme at 40 kilowatts. Because the National Programme used shorter wavelengths (higher frequencies) the range was somewhat less than that of the Regional Programme on 356 metres, however the long wave transmitter at Daventry also transmitted the National Programme and would fill in any areas of poorer reception. The BBC ensured that the new transmission arrangements would provide strong reception for listeners with both valved radios and humble crystal sets that were still being used.

Some transmitters also carried the BBC National Programme on a local frequency to supplement the long wave broadcasts from Daventry, Scotland received an amended service known as the 'Scottish National Programme'.

On September 6th 1934, the BBC opened a new Twin Wave station situated near the town of Droitwich to serve the Midlands region. Droitwich was to replace the existing transmitting site at Daventry. Initially the 5XX service used powerful new transmitters that produced 150 kilowatts. Five months later, on February 17th 1935, 5GB opened from Droitwich radiating the Regional Programme on medium wave with a power of 50 kilowatts and the original 5GB 25 kilowatt transmitter at Daventry was phased out.

Eventually further high power 'Twin Wave' stations would be built at Moorside Edge (North), Washford Cross (West) and Westerglen (Scottish). Additional high power transmitting stations were also established at Lisnagarvey, Burghead, Clevedon and Start Point to bring a Regional Programme to most areas of the UK. Additionally Penmon and Redmoss carried lower powered transmissions of the Welsh and Scottish regional programmes.

John Reith had been eager to provide an overseas radio service since 1924 and finally, after technical and financial delays, a licence to broadcast on short wave was acquired from the Post Office in 1926. The trial station G5SW opened at Chelmsford in November 1927. It was intended that G5SW would transmit programmes from Britain to the Empire from a 10 kW transmitter.

Short wave signals can travel thousands of miles across international boundaries by bouncing off the turbulent gases of the ionosphere, the layers of electrified gas high above the earth. However it's a signal that can be somewhat capricious - subject to interference from electrical storms and other atmospheric disturbances

The G5SW short wave transmissions were deemed to be a success and this led to the establishment of a permanent Empire Station at Daventry in December 1932 using two 15 kW transmitters and a number of directional aerial arrays to beam the signals to various parts of the globe.

The Empire Service was aimed principally at English speakers in the colonies of the British Empire, or as George V put it in the first-ever Royal Christmas Message, the "men and women, so cut off by the snow, the desert, or the sea, that only voices out of the air can reach them". His speech was scripted by the famous author Rudyard Kipling.

The Empire Service would expand in 1938. The first foreign language service was Arabic. A European service was started in the run up to the Second World War and French, German, Italian, Portuguese and Spanish were added.

The BBC took full advantage of emerging technology. Before 1930, the corporation had no viable means of recording sound. The first recording machine the BBC used was the Blattnerphone, which took its name from its inventor - early British filmmaker Louis Blattner. The Blattnerphone used 6mm steel tape to record a very basic audio signal that was good enough for voice recording but not for music. The machine's spools were large and heavy and editing was achieved by soldering the tape. The machine ran the tapes at a speed of 5 feet per second, which meant it was hazardous for the operator - a break in the tape could result in razor-edged steel flying around the studio.

There had been developments in microphone technology too. The AXBT was the 4th generation design of the original Marconi Type A microphone The ribbon microphone was particularly good in studio situations and the double-sided design, which accepted sound from front and back, but not from the side, was particularly suited to voice. It also gave the microphone its characteristic shape, which has entered popular culture as a symbolic image of broadcasting

By the end of the 1920s the premises at Savoy Hill were becoming inadequate for the BBC's needs. The heavy soundproofing drapes and lack of ventilation made it uncomfortable to broadcast there and a few performers fainted because of the heat.

The corporation had to find and establish a new operating centre. Initially a search was made for an existing building which could be adapted for the needs of broadcasting. After looking at several perties, including Dorchester House, which would subsequently be rebuilt as a hotel, it was decided that the problems of adaptation were too great and that it would be better, despite the greater expense, to construct a new building.

Various central London sites were considered and preliminary plans were prepared for some of them. Early in 1928 a site at the corner of Portland Place and Langham Street was proposed to the BBC. It was in the hands of a syndicate who were originally planning to build high-class residential flats. They offered to erect a building to suit the BBC's requirements and to grant a long-term lease, with an option to buy. An agreement between the BBC and the syndicate was signed on 21st November 1928. Incidentally the original lease barred certain tradesmen from the site, including slaughter men, sugar-bakers and brothel keepers.

George Val Myer designed the famous and now iconic Broadcasting House in collaboration with the BBC's civil engineer, M T Tudsbery. The interiors are the work of the Australian-Irish architect Raymond McGrath. He supervised a team that included Serge Chermayeff and Wells Coates. They designed the studio theatre, the associated green and dressing rooms, and the dance and chamber music studios in a flowing Art Deco style.

The architects faced the classic problem of a radio building - shielding the studios from extraneous noise. They decided to place all the offices in the form of an outer shell surrounding an inner core containing the studios. The offices consequently provided sound insulation for the studios.

The outer shell was constructed around a steel structure but there was still the problem of internal sound insulation. Steel would transmit sound from studio to studio so the central core was planned as a totally separate building within the outer shell. The central section was constructed almost entirely of brick.

Four separate plants provided air conditioning. Sound absorbing material was placed in the ventilation system to avoid sound travelling through the ducts. It was the first building in London to have artificially ventilated toilets. When completed, the building featured 22 studios, one mile of corridors, 1250 stairs, 800 doors and 50 miles of electrical wiring.

At the front of the building are statues designed by Eric Gill. The statues illustrate Prospero and Ariel from Shakespeare's 'The Tempest'. Their choice was fitting since Prospero was a magician, and Ariel, a spirit of the air, in which radio waves travel.

Construction was completed in 1931 and programmes transferred gradually to the new building. The first musical programme to be broadcast from Broadcasting House featured Henry Hall and his Dance Orchestra on March 15th 1932. Stuart Hibberd read the first news bulletin on March 18th. The last transmission from Savoy Hill was on May 14th 1932.

The total cost of building Broadcasting House was £500,000 and it was initially rented to the BBC at £45,000 p.a. It was later purchased for £650,000 and the freehold transferred to the BBC on 16 July 1936.

Despite all the planning, there were soon complaints about the facilities. The requirements of broadcasting had increased in the time it had taken to plan and build. Some studios were considered too small, doors were too narrow to allow equipment through and there was inadequate lighting to read scripts and scores.

Even with the efforts made by the architects, there was noise leakage between studios. The Concert Hall organ could be heard in other studios and conversely big bands playing in the sub-basement could be heard in the Concert Hall. The rumble of underground trains could be heard in the lower studios.

The total number of BBC employees doubled in the period between 1932 and 1936 and the Empire Service made demands on space and recording facilities. St. George's Hall, situated next door to the Queen's Hall, was acquired in 1933. It opened as a studio on November 25th, 1933 and was mainly used for music and variety shows. The BBC installed the original BBC Theatre Organ in 1936, a Compton Melotone and Electrostatic Organ. This enabled a wide range of sounds to be produced during performances. Reginald Foort was appointed resident organist.

A space suitable for large orchestras was required so an old ice-rink in Maida Vale was converted into a seven-studio complex in 1934. The 'Maida Vale Roller Skating Palace and Club' was built in 1909. Over a period of fifteen months, a team of one hundred men reduced the skating rink to a shell, and then proceeded to rebuild it. The outside structure of the building and the arches at the doorway were preserved. The BBC Symphony Orchestra moved here when the building was reopened and it has remained their base ever since.

Although the Maida Vale building has a drama studio, it's been chiefly used for recording musical sessions. Many famous musicians have recorded there from Big Bands to the Beatles. During World War II, Maida Vale served as the centre of BBC news operations throughout Europe. Much later Maida Vale became the home of the celebrated Radiophonic Workshop, which produced experimental electronic music for radio and television.

Sheila Barrett, the first female radio announcer, made her debut on July 28th 1933. Variety, or light entertainment as it was called at the BBC, was immensely popular in the thirties. However strict rules were introduced to ensure that there were no jokes about religion, drunkenness and many other sensitive subjects. Detailed guidelines were given to artists and producers and any act that breached them would have been severely reprimanded.

The most popular show of the 1930s was Band Waggon. The show only ran for a total of 55 episodes, but it had an enormous impact. Its memorable signature tune, extravagant musical items and irreverent humour made it pre-war radio's biggest success. However Band Waggon, as the name might suggest, hadn't actually been devised as a comedy programme. It was to be another dance band show but the BBC decided to broaden the shows appeal by adding a resident comedian and compere.

Richard Murdoch was chosen straight away as the compere. He was a song and dance man with a background in musical revue. The choice of resident comedian was more problematic. The producers couldn't choose between Tommy Trinder and Arthur Askey so a coin was tossed to decide which one of them should get the job - Heads for Trinder, tails for Askey. Heads won but as it turned out Tommy Trinder was unavailable. Therefore Arthur Askey was invited to join the show.

The first three shows were broadcast starting on 5th January 1938 but they were a disaster. The scriptwriter was fired and a scriptwriting team of Gordon Crier, Vernon Harris, Arthur Askey and Richard Murdoch took over. Arthur Askey and Richard Murdoch soon came to dominate the show and the musical parts were reduced.

The events and characters largely existed in the minds of the listeners. Many of their sketches had Arthur and Richard sharing a top floor flat in Broadcasting House along with Lewis the goat, and pigeons named Basil, Lucy, Ronald and Sarah. Other regular characters were Nausea Bagwash (Arthur's fictitious girlfriend) and her mother. These characters were often referred to but never heard.

The duo's adventures often ended violently with the famous Band Waggon crash. A corner of the stage was roped off and a large stack of assorted objects were piled up inside. At the appropriate moment it was pushed over by a sound effects man.

By the third series, Arthur Askey was in great demand for films and stage shows and Richard Murdoch had joined the RAF. Therefore it was decided to curtail the series after eleven shows. The last show was broadcast on December 2nd 1939 and Arthur and Richard departed from their famous flat for the final time.

The death of King George V in 1936 was an early milestone for the BBC newsroom and the subsequent state funeral was the first to be broadcast live. Later that year, the Abdication Crisis gripped Britain as King Edward VIII renounced the throne to marry the American divorcee Wallis Simpson.

The King's abdication speech was broadcast from Windsor Castle on December 10th 1936. Sir John Reith introduced the broadcast after giving Edward a voice test. Reith asked the outgoing monarch to read some text from the sports pages of a newspaper. Reith's diaries reveal that during the handover, Edward bumped the table at which he was seated. An audible thump was heard and this led some listeners to think Reith had left the room and slammed the door.

The BBC looked to expand its services and move into television. John Logie Baird, a Scottish engineer and inventor had been developing the world's first working television system since 1923. In 1932, the BBC began experimental television transmissions using the 30-line Baird system. These experiments emanated from studio BB in the basement of Broadcasting House.

In June 1935 the BBC installed a mast, studio and television transmitter at Alexandra Palace and continued experiments using two systems. John Logie Baird's electromechanical system had developed into a 240-line system at this point. It was alternated with an electronic scanning system developed jointly by EMI and Marconi. The Baird system, although similar in picture quality, proved troublesome for actors, directors, and other staff to use in the studio.

The world's first regular television service started on November 2nd 1936. The opening show was called 'Variety' and it's estimated that only 400 'lookers in' were able to see it. The musical comedy star Adele Dixon sang a song called simply 'Television' - known universally today as 'The Television Song'. It had been specially written for the occasion, with lyrics by James Dyrenforth and music by Kenneth Leslie-Smith.

Many ambitious outside broadcasts were made, including King George VI's coronation on May 12th 1937. About 10,000 people saw this on television. Other important landmarks included the first Wimbledon coverage in June 1937 and the F.A Cup Final in 1938.

The Television Advisory Committee eventually recommended that the BBC adopt the 405-line Marconi-EMI system in January 1937. Viewers were treated to a wide variety of programmes, including plays, newsreels, concerts, opera, ballet, cabaret and children's cartoons. The first three television presenters were Leslie Mitchell, Elizabeth Cowell and Jasmine Bligh. Leslie Mitchell was an ex actor whose handsome looks, smart suits and urbane public school manner endeared him to a nation. Elizabeth Cowell was tall, elegant and artistic. Jasmine Bligh was attractive, humorous and could improvise easily. It's been alleged that the cameramen would put gauze over their camera lenses to soften the beautiful Miss Bligh's looks if she had been to a party the previous night.

Pre-war television actors were paid considerably less than their radio counterparts. The BBC gave two reasons for this. The first reason seemed perfectly valid as television had a smaller audience. However the second was quite bizarre, the BBC reasoned that the actors should receive a reduced payment because they were shown in miniature.

John Reith disliked television intensely and was not even present at the public opening of the television service in 1936. By the mid 1930s, Reith's authoritarian style had many detractors. In an age of dictators it was easy to make comparisons. When Reith took his mother to tea at the House of Commons, the MP Nancy Astor asked if he got his 'Mussolini traits' from her.

Reith's own remarks didn't help. He said he respected Mussolini and talked in 1939 of Hitler's 'magnificent efficiency'. He also had a high regard for the German broadcasters: 'Germany has banned hot jazz and I'm sorry that we should be behind in dealing with this filthy product of modernity".

Throughout this period Reith was subjected to a media campaign criticising his managerial style. In 1934 Reith appeared in front of the 1922 Committee of Conservative MPs. Reith was able to present a petition signed by 800 BBC employees affirming their support.

For a man accused of being aloof from his workforce it is surprising to learn that he regularly took part in theatre productions by the staff amateur dramatic company. His last performance was in 1936 playing a butler in a play performed at the Fortune Theatre in London.

John Reith left the corporation on June 30th 1938. Reith left Broadcasting House for the last time without ceremony but he did carry out one more duty. Along with his secretary and his deputy Cecil Graves, they drove to the BBC transmitter at Droitwich in Worcestershire to switch it off at midnight. He signed the visitor's book 'J.C.W. Reith, late BBC'.

By the time the Second World War came, the BBC's five services (National, Regional, Overseas, Empire and Television) formed the nucleus of the greatest broadcasting company the world had ever seen.

5

Radio in America

On April 15th 1919, the American government ended the wartime ban on public reception of radio signals. This, together with improvements in vacuum-tube equipment, encouraged a number of private enterprises to be set up. The Chicago Radio Laboratory developed a 'Jeweller's Time Receiving Set'. This set received time signals transmitted by a number of Government Naval Radio Stations. In 1921, a catalogue from the William B. Duck Company offered a 'Type RS-100 Jeweller's Time Receiver' that promised to be an "exceptional commercial value to the jeweller since the time signals may be heard all over his store, and should produce an excellent advertisement for his business".

In early 1919, the U.S.S. George Washington had a valve transmitter installed for a transatlantic voyage. This was ostensibly to test long range radiotelephony but they still found time to broadcast occasional concerts. One of the ship's passengers was U.S. President Woodrow Wilson. It was announced that the president's Independence Day speech would be broadcast from aboard ship. However Wilson's speech went unheard because he stood too far from the microphone.

On May 30th 1920, the Navy transmitted live from the field of an Army - Navy baseball game at Annapolis, Maryland. High-powered radiotelegraph stations then relayed the game worldwide. 8MT, an amateur station in Pennsylvania broadcast advance information regarding the Uniontown Speedway races. 1DF, an amateur station in Winchester, Massachusetts, transmitted concerts on weekday nights and Sunday afternoons. The Michigan Agricultural College regularly transmitted weather reports, crop reports and extracts from lectures on agricultural topics.

There was a cluster of stations in the San Francisco area. The most prominent, was Lee De Forest's experimental station 6XC, the "California Theatre station", which started in April 1920. 2XG in New York, Lee De Forest's experimental station, broadcast a report from a football game on November 18th 1919. The station was also offering a nightly news broadcast. 2XX, another New York station frequently broadcast entertainment programmes from Broadway.

The proliferation of broadcasting stations led to a broadcasting boom, which swept across the United States in early 1922. Enthusiastic amateurs ran a lot of these stations and the Department of Commerce became worried about the quality of the broadcasts. They introduced regulations that restricted public broadcasting to stations, which met the criteria of a newly created broadcast service classification.

Despite these new regulations, radio stations continued to proliferate and by the end of the year there were over 500 stations transmitting to cities and towns across the country. The tremendous growth of radio broadcasting saw the development of a wide variety of innovative program offerings. 'The Man in the Moon' treated children listening to WJZ in Newark, New Jersey, to evening readings.

Radio captured the public imagination and it was increasingly reflected in popular culture. Songwriters began to mention it in their lyrics. These songs included 'I Wish There Was a Wireless to Heaven', published in 1922. This was followed six years later by a considerably happier tune 'A Bungalow, a Radio and You'.

Not everyone was happy with the programme offerings. Writer Charles E. Duffie criticised "the indiscriminate competitive jumble of phonograph music, uninteresting lectures, and disguised advertising talks, which have, in part, made up many programmes". He suggested the federal government could provide a better selection of programming.

The broadcasting boom triggered a huge increase in radio related literature. Numerous books and articles were published to introduce this exciting new innovation to the general public. These publications included basic information along with explanations of technical terms like 'static' and 'interference'. There was a considerable amount of books aimed at the younger reader. A lot of these books featured radio superficially as a prop or plot device. One notable exception to this was the Allen Chapman "Radio Boys" books. The books provided the usual elements of children's fiction but they also contained comprehensive and accurate technical details.

In America, even after the rise of radio broadcasting, a few experimenters continued to try to develop another way to set up multi-programme audio services. A few European countries briefly experimented with radio receivers that only picked up specific paid-for stations. However, this proved difficult to implement and far too easy to circumvent. Early radio experimenters found that multiple low-power transmissions could be carried along telegraph, telephone or electrical wires to distant points. To receive these transmissions people had to be located along the line. In 1923, there was an early (and ultimately unsuccessful) attempt to set up a subscription-based 'wired radio' service in New York City. Over succeeding decades the basic idea has been developed into a wide variety of innovations, from audio services to Cable TV.

Most European countries would ultimately decide to set up broadcasting as a government monopoly and charge their citizens fees for listening licences. However the United States radio industry developed in a different manner.

American Marconi dominated the post war radio and communications industry. However, despite the name, the vast majority of the company's stake holding remained in European hands. The American Government wanted to avoid foreign control of U.S. international communications so they applied extensive pressure on the company to sell its operations to an American firm. American Marconi's assets were subsequently sold to General Electric, which used them to form the patriotically named Radio Corporation of America.

On its formation, The Radio Corporation of America instantly became the dominant U.S. radio firm. Trade advertisements proclaimed that RCA was "an all-American concern holding the premier position in the radio field". The new company planned to build a showcase international facility, Radio Central, at Rocky Point in Long Island. The plans included ten Alexanderson alternator-transmitters, surrounded by twelve huge antennas arrayed in spokes each approximately 2 kilometres long. However, only about 20% of the planned alternator facilities were ever built, because within just a couple of years the development of far more efficient short wave transmissions made the long wave alternator-transmitters obsolete.

RCA quickly moved into the developing broadcasting field. Its debut broadcast was transmitted on July 2nd 1921 with a heavyweight boxing championship match between Jack Dempsey and Georges Carpentier. The bout was broadcast by WJY, with a transcript of the fight commentary telegraphed to KDKA in Pittsburgh, for rebroadcast by that station. There was a distinct lack of radio receivers so the majority of listeners were in halls, where volunteer amateurs set up radio receivers. Each listener was charged an admission fee, which was donated to charity.

The Westinghouse Electric & Manufacturing Company, based in Pennsylvania, also became one of the radio industry's most prominent leaders. Westinghouse was a major, manufacturer of electrical appliances for the home and was the first company to widely market radio receivers to the general public.

On November 2nd 1920, they began a public broadcasting service designed to promote the sale of radio receivers. The inaugural broadcast featured election returns broadcast from the company's new East Pittsburgh station. For the first few days the East Pittsburgh broadcasts went out under the Special Amateur call sign of 8ZZ, after which it switched to KDKA. The new station began daily broadcasts of varied offerings, which proved increasingly popular. Westinghouse quickly set up three additional stations - WJZ in Newark, WBZ in Massachusetts and KYW in Chicago.

The set up of the large American Radio Networks was made possible by experiments undertaken by the American Telephone & Telegraph Company (AT&T). The introduction of valve or vacuum-tube amplification for telephone lines allowed them to experiment with sending speeches to distant audiences that listened over loudspeakers. These short-range experiments soon progressed to transcontinental proportions. On November 11th 1921, audiences in New York City's Madison Square Garden and San Francisco's Civic Auditorium simultaneously heard President Harding's Armistice Day speech at the National Cemetery in Arlington, Virginia.

AT&T's next step was to use the lines to interconnect radio stations. Their aim was to set up the first nationwide network of connected radio stations. They formally announced this on February 11th 1922, although early statements referred to the set up as a "chain" of stations, rather than a network. AT&T's plan was to introduce what they called 'toll broadcasting'. They intended to sell the airtime to interested parties or organisations. Advertising would support the resulting programmes. Initially AT&T found it very difficult to persuade customers to purchase radio airtime. Their first success was transmitted from WEAF on August 28th 1922. It was a 15-minute talk promoting a Queensboro Corporation apartment complex. It cost the advertiser $50 and recouped $27,000 in sales

Although that talk has often been called "the first-ever radio commercial", there is evidence that other stations had previously sold airtime to commercial buyers. In Jersey City, Frank V. Bremer reportedly leased his amateur station, 2IA, to two local newspapers for a series of broadcasts.

1XE in Massachusetts - the American Radio & Research Corp.'s (AMRAD) experimental station, allegedly received money for reading stories from the Little Folk's Magazine and Youth's Companion. Later, when AMRAD got a new licence and started to broadcast with the call sign WGI they started to sell airtime officially. They hired a salesman to sell 30 hours of programming a week at the rate of $1 per minute. Their first sponsored programme was by the Packard Motor Company of Boston. However, WGI's commercial operations were almost immediately suspended. It was uncertain whether this was due to the intervention of the local District Radio Inspector, or AT&T enforcing what it felt was an infringement of its patent rights.

AT&T originally thought its patent rights would give it a near-monopoly of U.S. broadcasting and that only they had the exclusive right to sell advertising over the airwaves. By the beginning of 1923, there were over 500 broadcasting stations in America and the phone company claimed that the vast majority of these were infringing its copyrights. At this point the phone company resigned itself to the situation. They declared that it would, for an appropriate fee, licence other stations to carry on-air advertising. However the hundreds of stations did not rush to buy a licence.

In 1924, AT&T filed a patent-infringement lawsuit against WHN in New York City, which was eventually settled out of court. At the time of this settlement, WHN management loudly complained about AT&T's supposed plan to "monopolise" radio. WHN claimed that AT&T's licence demands were stifling the growth of commercial broadcasts but actually all stations settling with the phone company were permitted to sell advertising. They also acquired access to AT&T's lines for remote broadcasts. At this point, the rest of the broadcasting stations followed WHN's lead and stations that wanted to remain on the air dutifully paid for AT&T patent licences.

By the mid-1920s, many broadcasting stations found themselves facing increasing financial strain. Stations were forced to buy better, and subsequently more expensive, equipment to adhere to government engineering standards. Music publishers sought royalty payments for all copyrighted music that was aired and entertainers started to demand payment for their performances. In addition to those payments there were the AT&T licence fees to consider. This led to more and more stations selling airtime. This funding system, private stations supported by on-air advertising, remains the most common method used in the United States to this day.

This willingness to let anybody hire airtime led to some strange broadcasts. WLTH in Brooklyn had a rather odd sponsor - a mysterious bearded old man who bought a minute of time daily to declare his love for someone. During his minute of airtime he would constantly repeat the phrase 'I love you!' over and over again. He never revealed who his mysterious lover was but, as long as he paid the money, the station didn't care.

After a couple of years, AT&T's "toll broadcasting" experiment finally began to produce substantial returns. Weekly network programs such as 'The Ever Ready Hour' greatly expanded advertiser interest and network billing. So the phone company pressed ahead with their national network.

AT&T initially intended to own all of the stations in the network but ultimately they didn't need to do this. During the broadcast boom of 1922, hundreds of companies and individuals went ahead and built broadcast stations of their own. The phone company would only need to build their own broadcasting stations in two cities: WBAY and WEAF in New York and WCAP in Washington D.C. Most of AT&T's network broadcasts originated from WEAF in New York City and so the network was generally called the 'WEAF Chain'. However, company circuit charts marked the inter-city telephone links in red pencil, so the chain of stations was also informally known as 'the red network'.

The three companies that comprised the 'radio group' - General Electric, Westinghouse, and the Radio Corporation of America responded by creating their own, smaller, network. This centred on WJZ in New York City. AT&T blocked the rival network from using telephone lines so they had to find some other way to link up stations. At first the Radio Group used leased telegraph wires but the lines were susceptible to atmospheric and other electrical interference. Then they tried to connect the stations using short wave radio links but this also fell short of sound quality requirements.

In May 1926, AT&T decided that it no longer wanted to run a radio network and transferred its network operations into a wholly owned subsidiary, the Broadcasting Company of America. Then, rather unexpectedly, the Broadcasting Company of America was sold to the Radio Group companies for $1 million. They immediately shut WCAP in Washington and merged its facilities with surviving station WRC.

At this point a new company was formed, the National Broadcasting Company. This new organisation took over the Broadcasting Company of America assets and merged them with the radio group's fledgling network operations. The new division was divided in ownership between RCA (fifty percent), General Electric (thirty percent) and Westinghouse (twenty percent). NBC was officially launched on November 15th 1926.

AT&T's original WEAF Chain was officially renamed the NBC-Red network and the small network that the radio group had organized became the NBC-Blue network. The Red Network offered commercially sponsored entertainment and music programming. The Blue Network mostly carried sustaining or non-sponsored broadcasts such as news and cultural programmes.

On April 5th 1927, NBC reached the West Coast with the launch of the NBC Orange Network. This carried Eastern Red Network programming specially recreated for the West Coast. The NBC Gold Network made its debut on October 18th 1931 and carried programmes from the Blue Network. The Orange Network was dropped in 1936 and affiliate stations were incorporated into either the Blue or Red Networks. NBC also developed a network for short wave radio stations in the 1930s called the NBC-White Network.

Prior to 1927, radio was regulated by the United States Department of Commerce. Herbert Hoover, who was then Commerce Secretary, was highly influential in the shaping of American radio. Despite his important position, Hoover's powers were limited and he couldn't refuse a broadcasting licence to anyone who requested one. This resulted in too many stations trying to be heard on too few frequencies. After several failed attempts to rectify this situation, Congress finally passed the Radio Act of 1927. This legislation transferred the administration of radio to a newly created Federal Radio Commission (FRC), although some technical tasks remained the responsibility of the Department of Commerce's Radio Division.

The Federal Radio Commission was given the power to grant and deny licences. They also allocated frequencies and power levels for each licensee. The FRC was not given any official power of censorship, although programming could not include 'obscene, indecent, or profane language'. However the FRC's ability to revoke a broadcaster's licence or issue a fine obviously gave them a certain degree of control.

Many critics saw broadcasting regulation as an infringement of the First Amendment to the United States Constitution stating that the government shall not stop freedom of speech in the media. The FRC was extremely fastidious in its attempts to quash vulgar language, non-mainstream political views and "fringe" religions.

Almost immediately, the commission was accused of bias towards large commercial radio broadcasters at the expense of smaller non-commercial broadcasters. In reality, the FRC had virtually no control of the radio networks that were in the process of dominating U.S. radio. The networks were hardly mentioned in the Radio Act of 1927. The only reference was vague: The Commission shall "Have the authority to make special regulations applicable to stations engaged in chain broadcasting." The act did not permit the Federal Radio Commission to introduce any rules regulating advertising. The act merely required advertisers to be identified clearly within the broadcast

Early in 1928, the commissioners instigated a radical reorganisation of available frequencies. They forced 164 stations to justify their existence or they would be forced to stop broadcasting. Many low-powered independent stations were eliminated at this time, although eighty-one stations did survive, albeit with reduced power.

KFKB in Kansas was one of the most popular stations in America. The stations owner was a controversial medical doctor called John R. Brinkley. He regularly advocated the use of his own 'alternative' medications on air. He regularly recommended transplantation of goat glands into humans as a means of curing male impotence. In 1930 the Federal Radio Commission denied his request for renewal. Undeterred, he simply beamed his programmes to the United States from the powerful Mexican station XER.

XER was the first of many powerful Mexican stations to aim its programmes northwards. These stations, known as 'border blasters', could be heard over large areas of the U.S. They were also referred to as 'X Stations' for their call letters: Mexican stations are assigned call signs beginning with XE or XH, whereas American stations begin with the letters W or K. Canadian stations begin with C or VO.

The Mexican stations didn't have to adhere to U.S. broadcast laws and often passed themselves off as American. They would even disguise the fact by using a Texas post office box as a mailing address. The more unscrupulous stations, unfettered by the constraints of U.S. regulations, were free to peddle dubious goods. One such station hawked prayer handkerchiefs. They claimed these handkerchiefs negated the need for a doctor, as they would cure any ailment. Another radio evangelist reportedly was trying to sell listeners autographed photos of Jesus Christ.

During the 1930s radio technology had improved to such an extent that simultaneous global broadcasting became possible. In June 1930 General Electric engineers beamed a popular song, "I Love You Truly," around the world via short wave relays and rebroadcasts. They followed that feat with a radio bridge game between a team in New York and one in Argentina. However the most interesting stunt broadcast was a transmission between GE engineers in America and Australia. In New York they twisted a cat's tail and it meowed into a microphone. A dog at a loudspeaker in Australia heard the cat and barked into a microphone. Back in New York the cat responded by arching its back and ruffling its fur - thus completing the world's first transoceanic dog-and-cat fight.

As the big networks expanded many independently owned radio stations applied to join them. The stations that carried network programming were termed as affiliates. These affiliates agreed to carry designated network programs. Since the programs included commercials, the stations received a share of the network revenue. At the same time, the affiliates could run their own local commercials around the network programmes.

Between 1930 and the mid 1950s, NBC was the dominating force in American radio. The network's stations were frequently the most powerful in their area. Many broadcast on clear frequencies that were capable of transmitting hundreds or thousands of miles at night. However the main reason behind NBC's popularity had to be the programmes that were transmitted during this period. American radio's earliest mass hit was broadcast by NBC. Amos 'n' Andy began in 1926–27 as a fifteen-minute serial. The two struggling title characters appealed to a broad audience, especially during the Great Depression.

NBC became home to many of the most popular performers and programmes on the air. Bob Hope, Al Jolson, Burns and Allen, Jack Benny, Edgar Bergen and Fred Allen were all mainstays of the network. Popular programmes included The Great Gildersleeve, Vic and Sade, One Man's Family, Death Valley Days, Ma Perkins, and Fibber McGee and Molly.

The famous three-note NBC chimes evolved after several years of development. The chimes were first heard on WSB in Atlanta. Someone at NBC in New York heard the three note sequence during the networked broadcast of a Georgia Tech football game and asked permission to use it on the national network. NBC started to use the three notes in 1931 and were mechanized in 1932. They were used as a cue for switching different stations between the Red and Blue network feeds.

The NBC chimes were the first audio trademark to be accepted by the U.S. Patent and Trademark Office. Contrary to popular legend, the three musical notes, G-E'-C', did not stand for the General Electric Company. General Electric was forced to sell its share of RCA in 1930 because of antitrust charges. A variant sequence, known as "the fourth chime, was used during wartime and in time of disasters.

NBC's main rival was the Columbia Broadcasting System. CBS began as United Independent Broadcasters with 16 affiliates. When Columbia Records invested in the radio network in 1927, it became the Columbia Phonographic Broadcasting System. The Paley family, who owned a tobacco firm, secured majority ownership of the network in 1928. The name was streamlined to the Columbia Broadcasting System at this point

Samuel Paley's intention had been to use his acquisition as nothing more than an advertising medium for promoting the family business. This proved a shrewd move as cigar sales more than doubled after a year. The new owners soon found that they could sell far more than just cigars over the airwaves. Sam Paley faced increased demands on his time so handed control of the radio network to his 26-year old son William S. Paley. Within a decade, under Bill Paley's inspired leadership, the CBS network expanded to 114 affiliate stations with WCAU as the flagship station.

Paley built his empire by sweet-talking the very best performers and technical talent of the era to join CBS; Paley brazenly stole shows and performers from competing networks and his relentless pursuit of the best talent in the industry paid dividends for his network.

CBS were at the heart of an event that became known as the press-radio war. Like their European counterparts, the American newspapers saw radio as a serious competitor. The major news services, including the Associated Press (AP), the International News Service (INS), and the United Press (UP), launched a battle against the radio stations. The agencies threatened to cut off radio's flow of news. The newspaper groups could do this by restricting access to teletype machines. The teletypes supplied the country's newspapers with regular summaries of news, feature stories, weather forecasts and bulletins.

Recognizing the consequences of this threat, CBS set up their own news gathering agency. This enraged the newspaper groups who issued a list of demands. The first demand was the total cessation of CBS's news gathering operations. They also tried to restrict the amount of news broadcasts to two news summaries a day, which could only be aired after the morning and afternoon newspapers were published. They further stipulated that the newscasts could not be sponsored. CBS eventually won the battle and proceeded to assemble the one of the most respected and knowledgeable news teams in the history of radio broadcasting.

Radio stations gradually reduced their commitments to news. They realised that news gathering was hugely expensive. Ratings also indicated that most listeners were more interested in hearing entertainment than news. Nowadays most American stations switch to an audio network on the hour for a short news summary

CBS radio produced dozens of long running shows. One of the most fondly remembered shows is 'Suspense' which ran from 1942 to 1962. The programme was subtitled "radio's outstanding theatre of thrills," and focused on suspense thriller-type scripts, usually featuring leading Hollywood actors of the era. Approximately 945 episodes were broadcast during its long run.

CBS were responsible for the most infamous broadcast in American radio history. On the evening of October 30th 1938, The Mercury Theatre's adaptation of H.G.Wells' science fiction tale, 'The War of the Worlds' caused widespread mayhem. Rather than a straightforward dramatic adaptation of the novel about an alien invasion from Mars, Orson Welles chose to portray the events in the book differently. He changed the location and time from Victorian England to contemporary America. More importantly, the first half of the story was presented as a simulated broadcast with mock news bulletins and on the spot reports. It was undoubtedly this novel dramatic device that led to the subsequent panic.

Writer Howard Koch chose Grover's Mill as the location for the first Martian landing by randomly prodding a pencil into a map. He then plotted the Martians route toward New York City, defeating the army and destroying dozens of familiar place names along the way. Unfortunately listeners tuning in late had absolutely no idea that what they were experiencing was a dramatic presentation. In the programme makers' defence, the show was clearly advertised as such. There were also several clear announcements before, during, and after the broadcast that clearly stated that the show was a dramatization of H.G.Wells short story.

Nevertheless, many listeners thought the broadcast was fact, not fiction. People fled their homes in terror, carried weapons in an attempt to defend themselves against aliens and even wrapped their heads in wet towels as protection from Martian poison gas. CBS stations, city authorities and police forces around the country received hundreds of telephone calls from panic-stricken listeners.

News of the panic quickly generated a national scandal. In the days following the adaptation there was widespread anger towards the perpetrators. The program's news-bulletin format was condemned as maliciously deceptive by some newspapers. Gradually the chorus of disapproval subsided and many public figures spoke out in favour of the broadcast. In a perceptive column, in the New York Tribune, Dorothy Thompson stated that the broadcast exposed how politicians could utilize the media to create theatrical illusions and manipulate the public.

The Mutual Broadcasting System operated from 1934 to 1999. Of the four national networks during American radio's classic era, the MBS had the largest number of affiliates. Despite this, the network was constantly in a precarious position financially. For the first eighteen years of its existence, MBS was owned and operated as a cooperative. Unlike NBC and CBS, which distributed programs to affiliated stations, the original Mutual was an arrangement among its four founding stations to share programmes produced at the stations.

Mutual's original participating stations were WOR in New Jersey, WGN in Chicago, WXYZ located in Detroit and Cincinnati's WLW. As they were located in the two largest markets, WOR and WGN provided the bulk of the programming. WXYZ left Mutual in 1935 and was replaced by CKLW in Ontario Canada.

The MBS struggled to make ends meet in its early years. In 1935, the cooperative only sold $1.1 million dollars in advertising. Compare that amount to the $26.6 million in sales logged by NBC and $16.3 million achieved by CBS that same year. It was only when the Colonial and Don Lee regional networks were amalgamated into the network in 1936 that MBS achieved national coverage. In 1947, Mutual had 400 affiliates and that figure had risen to 560 by 1952. At this point, the General Tire Company purchased the network and its days as a co-operative were over. After this the MBS was purchased by a succession of conglomerates including Armand Hammer, The Hal Roach Studios and 3M.

MBS's shaky financial position influenced the type of programming it aired. Entertainment and music shows were expensive to produce so Mutual aired a lot of low-budget dramatic shows. Most of these shows were produced at WOR, using a repertory company of New York actors. 'The 'Mysterious Traveller' is a fine example of the types of show produced. Children's serials were also relatively cheap to produce. 'Red Ryder' and 'The Adventures of Superman' generated a lot of revenue for the network. Sport was another lucrative money earner for Mutual. For many years it broadcast commentaries on major sporting events such as the Baseball World Series and Notre Dame Football.

Despite limited resources MBS produced some of the best programmes of the era. 'Sherlock Holmes', 'Dick Tracy', 'The Green Hornet and 'The Shadow' were all big hits on the network. The latter programme is arguably the most fondly remembered show of the period.The Shadow was undoubtedly the most popular crime show on the radio, often drawing as many as 15 million listeners.

The Shadow had been featured on the NBC and CBS network between 1930 and 1933 but this version had been a crime anthology series. In these early shows the Shadow served merely as the narrator. When he first appeared on the Mutual Network in 1937, the Shadow had been reinvented as a man of action. According to the show's introduction, The Shadow was, "in reality, Lamont Cranston, wealthy young man about town." Cranston had been taught a "strange and mysterious secret, the power to cloud men's minds so that they cannot see him." The Shadow used these powers of invisibility and hypnosis to solve crimes. Joining Cranston on his adventures was Margo Lane, his "friend and companion."

The Shadow had significant cast turnover throughout its seventeen year run on Mutual. Orson Welles, Bill Johnstone, Bret Morrison, John Archer and Steve Courtleigh all played the title character while a succession of actresses played Margo. These included Agnes Moorehead, Judith Allen, Laura Mae Carpenter, Grace Matthews, Marjorie Anderson, Lesley Woods and Gertrude Warner.

The episodes were largely formulaic and one of the most common themes revolved around the failures of scientific discovery. Villains were frequently scientists or intellectuals who used their research for evil rather than the benefit of mankind. Margot Lane was the stereotypical damsel in distress in most episodes, finding herself in the clutches of that week's villain. It was up to Cranston to save her without revealing his identity.

The 1930s through to the 1950s are often referred to as the 'Golden Age of Radio'. The broadcasts caught the public imagination. In 1933, 3.6 million radio sets were sold and this was during the Depression. By 1939 about 80 percent of Americans owned radios.

Radio borrowed much of its broadcast format from other entertainment media. During the 1930s, 'The Amos and Andy Show' was an astounding success. The programme harked back to an older entertainment tradition - the minstrel show. This was when white entertainers painted their faces black and pretended to be Negroes. Two white comedians, Freeman Gosden and Charles Correll, brought this dubious genre to radio. Nevertheless Amos and Andy were so popular that telephone use dropped 50 percent during their broadcasts and cinemas interrupted screenings to pipe in the programme.

Another unlikely radio success was ventriloquist act, Edgar Bergen and Charlie McCarthy. The popularity of a ventriloquist on radio, when nobody could see neither the dummy nor his skill, mystified many critics. It was Bergen's skill as an entertainer and vocal performer, and especially his characterization of Charlie that carried the show. Edgar and Charlie were continuously on the radio until 1956. Bergen's success on radio was paralleled in the United Kingdom by Peter Brough and his dummy Archie Andrews who featured in the BBC show 'Educating Archie'.

Music was also a principal source of programming for radio. Live symphonic orchestra performances were common, with CBS sponsoring broadcasts by the New York Philharmonic and NBC forming an orchestra around the talents of Italian maestro Arturo Toscanini. However the most popular music on radio came from the theatres and dance halls. Singers such as Bing Crosby, Ella Fitzgerald, Rudy Vallee and Dinah Shore became firm audience favourites.

Famous swing and jazz stars such as Benny Goodman, Louis Armstrong, Artie Shaw, Cab Calloway, Tommy Dorsey and Duke Ellington broadcast regularly. These transmissions were almost always live, as few records were licensed for radio broadcast. This was because a long-standing royalty dispute between broadcasters and the American Federation of Musicians and American Society of Composers, Authors and Publishers. The dispute effectively barred the use of recorded music on American radio.

Sports programmes became instantly popular. Baseball, boxing, and college football all proved successful in attracting audiences. The future American president Ronald Reagan was a sports announcer at WHO in Iowa during the 1930s and regularly commentated on baseball games by the Chicago Cubs. During away games Reagan remained in the Des Moines studio He was fed the raw data from the game by telegraph and invented the remainder of the action.

A more original staple of radio was the daily serial aimed largely at a female audience. These broadcasts became known as 'soap operas' because household-products advertisers, such as soap makers, usually sponsored them. The soaps served up daily doses of romance and melodrama to their enthusiastic audience. The first soap opera was 'The Romance of Helen Trent', which made its debut in 1933 and lasted until 1960. Other favourites included 'Just

Plain Bill', 'Our Gal Sunday', 'Backstage Wife' and 'Ma Perkins'.

The most popular dramas tended to be crime and suspense stories, occasionally drawn from contemporary comic books, pulp magazines and classic fiction. They included Charlie Chan, Tom Mix, Tarzan, Sherlock Holmes, Buck Rogers in the Year 2430 and Jack Armstrong, the All-American Boy. The horror anthology series was also fashionable. 'Lights Out' was a particularly gruesome example of this genre. Sound effects technicians would gleefully accentuate events happening within the drama with outlandish sounds. For example, they would produce the sound of splattering blood and guts by immersing a bathroom plunger in warm spaghetti.

At the beginning of the Golden Age, American radio network programmes were almost exclusively broadcast live. The national networks prohibited the airing of recorded programmes until the late 1940s. This was mostly due to the inferior sound quality of phonograph discs. As a result, prime-time shows would be performed twice, once for each coast. The reason why many of these shows survive today is because "reference recordings" were made as they were being broadcast. This would have been for review by the sponsor or for the network's own archival purposes. The pre recording of shows became more common after World War II, when high-fidelity magnetic wire and tape recording techniques were developed.

Local stations, however, had always been free to use recordings and sometimes made extensive use of prerecorded syndicated programmes. When a substantial number of copies of an electrical transcription were required they were produced by the same process used to make ordinary records. An electroplated master recording was cut, from which pressings in vinyl were moulded in a record press.

These recordings were made using a cutting lathe and acetate discs. Programmes were usually recorded at 33 1/3 rpm on 16 inch discs, the standard format used for such "electrical transcriptions" from the early 1930s through to the 1950s. Sometimes, the groove was cut starting at the inside of the disc and running to the outside. This was useful when the programme to be recorded was longer than 15 minutes so required more than one disc side. By recording the first side outside in, the second inside out, and so on, the sound quality at the disc change-over points would match and result in a more seamless playback.

An inside start also had the advantage that the thread of material cut from the disc's surface, which had to be kept out of the path of the cutting stylus, was naturally thrown toward the centre of the disc so was automatically out of the way. When cutting an outside start disc, a brush could be used to keep it out of the way by sweeping it toward the middle of the disc. Well-equipped recording lathes used the vacuum from a water aspirator to pick it up as it was cut and deposit it in a water-filled bottle. In addition to convenience, this served a safety purpose, as the cellulose nitrate thread was highly flammable and a loose accumulation of it combusted violently if ignited.

Most recordings of radio broadcasts were made at a radio network's studios, or at the facilities of a network-owned or affiliated station, which might have four or more lathes. A small local station often had none. Two lathes were required to capture a program longer than 15 minutes without losing parts of it while discs were flipped over or changed, along with a trained technician to operate them and monitor the recording while it was being made.

In the mid 1930s, American radio stations got a new regulatory body to oversee their development. In 1934, Congress passed the Communications Act, which abolished the Federal Radio Commission The new Federal Communications Commission took over the existing responsibilities of the FRC and also acquired jurisdiction over telephone and telegraph companies.

In 1939, the FCC thought that NBC's two networks gave it an unfair advantage over its competitors and ordered RCA to divest itself of one of the two networks. There followed a long legal battle but losing its final appeal before the U.S. Supreme Court in May 1943, RCA sold the Blue Network for $8 million to Edward J. Noble. The new owner also owned Life Savers candy and the Rexall drugstore chain

Noble wanted a better name for the network and in 1944 acquired the rights to the name American Broadcasting Company. The Blue Network became ABC officially on June 15th 1945. Therefore ABC and NBC, although bitter rivals nowadays, are essentially fraternal twins separated by a custody battle.

ABC was not an instant success and had to build an audience gradually. ABC did this by purchasing more stations. The most significant addition was the highly profitable Detroit station WXYZ. This station was where The Lone Ranger, Sergeant Preston and The Green Hornet originated, although these programmes were not included in the deal. Noble also bought KECA in Los Angeles and this gave the network a Hollywood production base. Although ABC was still in fourth place by the late 1940s, they began to gain ground on the better-established networks.

Alternative programming became an ABC specialty. They would broadcast a boisterous quiz-show like 'Stop the Music!' against more sedate offerings on the other networks. ABC was the first to utilise advances in tape-recording technology brought back from Europe. The new network pre-recorded many programmes as the audio quality of tape was equal to that of "live" broadcasts. Consequently ABC was able to attract several high-rated stars who wanted freedom from rigid schedules. Bing Crosby was probably the most high-profile star who joined ABC during this period.

After the Second World War, Sunday night became the main ratings period with all the networks jostling for the top spot. In the late 1940s, CBS gained ground by allowing radio stars to use their own production companies, which proved highly profitable for them. Jack Benny, the nation's top radio star at the time, was the first of many NBC performers to transfer to CBS.

NBC hit back with The Big Show in November 1950. This 90-minute variety show updated radio's earliest musical variety style with sophisticated comedy and dramatic presentations. It regularly featured prestigious entertainers such as Fred Allen, Louis Armstrong, Groucho Marx, Ethel Merman, Bob Hope and Ella Fitzgerald. The show's regular hostess was stage legend Tallulah Bankhead. However the Big Show's initial success didn't last, despite critical praise, as most of its potential listeners were increasingly watching television instead. The show limped on for two years before cancellation. It's estimated that NBC lost a million dollars on the project as they were only able to sell advertising time during the middle half-hour every week.

NBC's last major radio programming push of the golden era began on June 12th 1955. Monitor was a continuous all-weekend mixture of music, news, interviews and features. The programme was a success for several years but listening figures dipped during the 1960s. Local stations, especially in larger markets, were reluctant to break from their established formats to run non-conforming network programming. Very little remained of NBC network radio when Monitor finished its run on January 26th 1975. The only things left were hourly newscasts and news features.

The NBC News and Information Service was launched on June 18th 1975. This service provided up to 55 minutes of news per hour around the clock to local stations that wanted to adopt an all-news format. However the service failed to attract enough stations and was discontinued in 1977.

The end of the era now known in America as the 'Golden Age of Radio' is hard to pinpoint. Most people agree that it falls somewhere between 1957 and 1962 but there are several milestones that account for radio's gradual decline. In the late 1930s the royalty dispute between musicians and broadcasters was settled. This agreement led to more recorded music being transmitted and the end of live broadcasts of orchestras. The federal government was about to crack down on radio-station networks on the basis that they violated antitrust laws. Most important of all, at the 1939 New York World's Fair, the public was introduced to television. Although the Second World War would delay the deployment of this new technology, it signalled the end of radio's media dominance.

By the middle of the 1950s a lot of radio stars had transferred to television, and the networks focused their resources on the new visual medium. Radio audiences went into a steep decline and many popular programmes were axed. The final episodes of 'Yours Truly, Johnny Dollar' and 'Suspense' are often cited as the end of the golden age of radio in America. The last episode of 'Johnny Dollar' ended at 6:35 p.m. Eastern Time on September 30th 1962, followed immediately by the final broadcast of 'Suspense'. When these two radio favourites ended that gave a clear signal that the 'Golden Age' was well and truly over.

6

Voices From Europe

In 1922, the British Government awarded a monopoly broadcasting licence to a single British Broadcasting Company. This arrangement lasted until 1927, when the broadcasting licence of the original BBC was allowed to expire. The assets of the former commercial company were then sold to a new non-commercial British Broadcasting Corporation, which operated under a UK charter from the Crown. This meant there was no possibility of commercial broadcasters operating from inside the United Kingdom. The BBC undoubtedly provided quality programming of great broadcasting worth but some listeners found this type of programming dull and monotonous and looked for an alternative.

The early British wireless experimenters would often try to hear stations from the continent. This practice was called 'searching the ether'. An early favourite was the privately owned station PCGG in Holland. The station was run by Hans Idzerda to promote sales of his company's crystal sets and components.

The station evolved from a 'one-off' transmission in 1919. The broadcast's time, date and frequency were advertised in the press. The Programme was called 'Soiree Musicale' and transmitted from The Hague between 8.00pm and 11.00pm on the 6th November. Philips, the Dutch electrical firm, sponsored it. The broadcast reached an unexpectedly large audience and Idzerda was encouraged to introduce regular transmissions.

The station was useful to listeners in gauging the efficiency of their set. If they could pick up The Hague Sunday afternoon concert on 1070 metres then it was a good receiver. Concerts were also transmitted on Monday and Thursday evenings. Multilingual announcements were made in Dutch, French and English.

PCGG's broadcasts proved to be very popular and elicited a great deal of listener correspondence. Idzerda managed to secure sponsorship, some from as far afield as the United Kingdom. However Idzerda got into financial difficulties and his licence was withdrawn on November 11th 1924. His company was declared bankrupt a month later.

Nevertheless there were more commercial experiments throughout the 1920s. In 1925 Selfridge's in London sponsored a fifteen-minute fashion talk from a studio on the Eiffel Tower. In 1927 and 1928 the Kolster Brand radio manufacturer sponsored a string of English concerts by the De Groot Orchestra from Hilversum.

A rather unusual commercial radio venture took place in 1928. The Daily Mail newspaper group chartered a 'Broadcasting Yacht', which was an early forerunner of the 1960s 'pirate radio' ships. The idea was to broadcast at sea from just outside the three-mile limit and advertise the Daily Mail, the Evening News and the Sunday Dispatch.

They set off from Dundee with a small transmitter on board but soon encountered problems. They were only able to broadcast when the sea was calm and the idea of transmitting at sea was swiftly abandoned. The German firm of Siemens Halske offered a solution by supplying four super loudspeakers, each weighing 6 1/2 cwt, and mounting them on the yacht's superstructure. This public address system was capable of being heard clearly for more than two miles on a moderately clear day. They were able to continue their cruise around the coast of Britain, blasting out gramophone records and publicising their newspapers.

From 1929 to 1931, the Vocalion Record Company sponsored an occasional series of record programmes from Radio Toulouse. They were not the only record company to realise the potential of radio. Decca Records sponsored a programme on Radio Paris with both French and English announcers. The announcers would give the details of the record played and invite listeners' requests for the following programme.

The fashion talk aired from the Eiffel Tower in 1925 had been arranged by British entrepreneur Leonard F. Plugge. He was a former RAF Captain and engineer on the London Underground. Plugge was a radio enthusiast and listened intently to the continental stations. He even wrote a couple of articles about them for the Radio Times. He quickly became obsessed with the new medium, and its commercial possibilities.

Plugge pronounced his name "Plooje", claiming Belgian-Dutch origins. It was only when he later stood for parliament that he agreed to the slogan "Plugge in for Chatham" and accepted the way almost everybody else pronounced his name.

Plugge was a pioneer of long motoring holidays on the European continent. On one such journey he stopped for coffee at the Café Colonne in the coastal village of Fécamp in Normandy. He asked the café owner what there was to see in the town, and was told that a young member of the Le Grand family – which owned the town's Benedictine Distillery – had a small radio transmitter behind a piano in his house.

Always keen to meet another radio enthusiast, Plugge went to see Fernand Le Grand at his home. During their conversation Le Grand told Plugge that in one broadcast he mentioned the name of a local shoemaker and recommended his wares. The shoemaker's sales increased enormously. Plugge instantly saw the commercial possibilities and offered to buy time to broadcast programmes in English. Le Grand agreed and Plugge formed the International Broadcasting Company.

The fledgling organisation needed a base in London to handle advertising. So the IBC, as it became known, opened premises at 11 Hallam Street in London. The new headquarters were just a short distance away from the BBC's Broadcasting House, which was being built at the time.

A studio was set up in the hayloft over the old stables in Rue George Cuvier. Old rugs draped the walls and stable matting was placed on the floor to reduce any extraneous noise. The transmitter site was moved to the Benedictine Distillery's herb garden at the edge of the Normandy cliffs. The transmitter was housed a small hut and the signal was fed to two second-hand aerial masts. This set-up provided a strong signal heard throughout London and the South of England.

Radio Fécamp started broadcasting in English on September 6th 1931. IBC's English programmes were broadcast after the French programmes had gone off the air. The first presenter was a cashier from the National Provincial Bank's Le Havre branch, whom Plugge had met when drawing cash after leaving Le Grand. William Evelyn Kingwell agreed to motorcycle over on Sundays to introduce records. The programmes were broadcast between 10.30 to 1am.

Kingwell fell ill and Plugge brought in new announcers - Bob Danvers-Walker and Max Staniforth. The station became Radio Normandy at this point (the station used this anglicised spelling in its British literature and advertising). Programmes were transmitted every Saturday and Sunday.

Staniforth was an ex-army Major who was hired to be Plugge's 'man on the ground'. He moved his family to Fécamp and they would make guest appearances on air. Staniforth remained at Normandy until November 1932. He was transferred to Radio Toulouse before taking up a position at IBC's headquarters in London. Staniforth eventually left broadcasting to join the church.

Bob Danvers-Walker began his radio career in Melbourne, Australia, in 1925, moving on briefly to ABC in Sydney in 1932 before returning to join IBC that same year. He became Chief Announcer at Radio Normandy. He also helped set up radio stations at Paris, Madrid, Barcelona and Valencia.

Danvers-Walker went on to carve out a memorable career in broadcasting. He joined the BBC in 1943, and was deployed on a variety of morale-boosting wartime radio shows, including 'Round and About' and 'London Calling Europe'. In the 1950s Danvers-Walker was one of the regular presenters of 'Housewives' Choice' and contributed to many other programmes. He also worked for Radio Luxembourg and was the announcer for 'Much-Binding-In-The-Marsh' and the science-fiction series 'Dan Dare, Pilot of the Future'.

His rich, distinctive voice became familiar to cinemagoers as the anonymous off-screen commentator for the twice-weekly British Pathe newsreel, a job he held continuously from 1940 to 1970. The upbeat, patriotic, "stiff upper lip" style he adopted in this role soon became a kind of standard for the medium, and is still parodied to this day whenever television or film wants to suggest 1940s and 1950s news coverage. The arrival of commercial television to Britain in 1955 brought him many new opportunities, including the announcer on Michael Miles' popular networked game show Take Your Pick

Many others joined during the life of Radio Normandy. David Davies became General Manager and Chief Announcer. After the war

Davies held a similar role at Radio Lourenco Marques in South Africa.

David Newman joined the station in 1936. There was already a gentleman with the same name who worked for IBC so he became Ian Newman on air. Newman married a French Girl and stayed with the station until the outbreak of World War II. After the war Newman joined the Foreign Office in the Diplomatic Service

By April 1933, English programmes were being transmitted from Fécamp every day of the week. In an effort to gauge listenership, Radio Normandy set up the "International Broadcasting Club". It cost nothing to join, just the price of a stamp. Within three weeks nearly 50,000 applications had been received. Three months later months more than a quarter of a million names were on the membership list.

Radio Normandy could be heard across Southern England and beyond and its output swiftly became popular. The programmes were livelier than the stodgy BBC output. On Sundays, when the BBC was concentrating on religious output, Radio Normandy was said to command 80% of the British radio audience.

Radio Normandy was entirely financed by advertising. Philco was an early sponsor. Henleys, a car sales company, successfully launched the SS1 motorcar on the station. This proved to sceptics that radio advertising really worked. Henley's went on to become a chain of car showrooms and repair garages from which later Jaguars, Rovers, Land Rovers etc, were sold. While SS Cars, also known as Swallow Sidecars, went on to become Jaguar Cars!

At the other end of the spectrum, companies who produced affordable goods aimed at the household or medicinal markets also invested heavily. Vitamin pills, nerve tonics and mouthwashes were offered to combat such conditions such as `body odour', `halitosis', `listlessness', `night starvation' and `tell-tale tongue'.

Normandy's programmes were expanded in 1932 and ran from 6pm to 3am. The power of the transmitter increased after Plugge received backing from film studio and cinema chain owner Gaumont British. A new studio was established in a house in the town. Radio Normandy by now had a large audience as far north as the English Midlands, and many big names of the day were heard. Among them was Roy

Plomley, later famous for creating and presenting Desert Island Discs for BBC radio.

Roy Plomley took charge of an increasingly important part of the IBC Empire – outside broadcasts. The best remembered of these was 'Radio Normandy Calling'. This was a touring review that first appeared in March 1938. Sponsored by Maclean's Peroxide Toothpaste, Radio Normandy Calling presented acts such as Alfredo and his Gypsy Band, Ward and Draper (singers), Maisie Weldon (impressionist) and Joe Young (comedian).

The organisation had a fleet of trucks that traversed the country recording specially staged variety shows from cinemas and theatres. These performances were cut onto wax discs using bulky and primitive equipment aboard each van.

The recording machine, or 'lathe' as it was often referred to, was a larger version of a typical gramophone of the time with a heavy metal base. Each machine had an extremely cumbersome electric motor at the back. A special type of cutting head replaced the typical pick-up arm of a record player. The cutting head was simply a phonograph pickup in reverse; audio was fed in and transferred to the disc on the turntable. The cutting head was moved uniformly across the radius of the disc by means of a slowly rotating feed screw mechanism.

The wax discs were big and heavy and could only be played back once. The method of playback also damaged the discs considerably. Copies could be made but this was a very costly practice. Luckily a new development was available that made the process easier and more reliable. Cecil Watts, a musician turned inventor, invented the lacquer-coated disc. An aluminium or glass disc was layered with a cellulose-nitrate lacquer. These discs were tough enough to playback several times without wearing out. Unfortunately the chemical composition of the lacquer has ensured that only a few of these discs survive today.

The International Broadcasting Company began leasing airtime from other radio stations in Europe and reselling it as sponsored English language programming aimed at audiences in Britain and Ireland. The IBC established a network of stations broadcasting sporadically across the continent.

Radio Toulouse started English broadcasts in October 1931 with W Brown Constable at the helm. The first programme was 'The Vocalion Concert Of Newly Released Records'. Brown Constable lasted until 1933 when Tom Ronald replaced him. Ronald's tenure at Toulouse was brief when broadcasting was suspended in July of that year.

When English broadcasts resumed in 1937, it was with a different company. The advertising agency WED Allen was run by three brothers who struck up a relationship with Peter Eckersley, the eccentric ex BBC and Marconi engineer. The inaugural programme featured a speech by Winston Churchill. The main on air personalities were Joslyn Mainprice, Allan Rose and Polly Ward.

Programmes included Feen-a-Mint Fanfare, Horlicks Picture House and the Empire Pools Sports programme. The station failed to attract enough advertising and folded in May 1938.

Radio Cote D'Azur was established in April 1934. English programmes were transmitted from 10.30 pm every Sunday night. The programmes consisted mainly of gramophone records introduced by Leo Bailet. However there were regular transcribed relays from the 'Sporting Club' in Monte Carlo and the 'Coconut Grove' in Hollywood.

In 1935, the French Government announced plans to transmit from Nice and call the station Radio Cote D'Azur They demanded that the commercial station changed its name. The station dutifully changed its name to Radio Mediterranee and this incarnation lasted until January 1938.

Radio Rome's first English broadcast was 'A Concert of Mayfair Records' sponsored by Ardath Cigarettes. Alexander Wright was the IBC announcer. Italy was not one of IBC's successes and English shows only lasted for a couple of months until October 1934.

The Spanish stations lasted longer. The IBC began to hire time on Radio Valencia, Radio Barcelona, Radio San Sebastian and Union Radio Madrid. H. Gordon Box and Bob Danvers Walker shared the announcing duties. Programmes started in December 1933 and lasted until March 1935. Broadcasts from these stations ended because of the worsening political situation that eventually led to the Spanish Civil War in 1936.

English programming on Poste Parisien started off in a small way. In 1934, English shows were broadcast for only four hours per month. However by 1939 this had expanded to eighteen hours per week. This may have been at the instigation of Douglas Pollock. In addition to his duties as the main announcer, he was also a director of Poste Parisien. IBC were appointed as the main contractor and a lot of familiar sponsored shows were transmitted. Poste Parisien's 'state of the art' facilities included a large concert hall and two smaller studios. Station announcements were punctuated by the sound of a gong being struck. Radio Luxembourg would also adopt this practice much later.

If a station was closed down another would pop up in its place. IBC programmes were also broadcast from Radio Ljubljana in Yugoslavia and Irish stations such as Dublin, Cork and Athlone. The IBC stations had 21 advertising sponsors in 1932. By 1935, annual revenue had climbed to £400,000 and that figure had risen to £1,700,000 in 1938.

An IBC announcer tended to lead a peripatetic lifestyle as they were transferred to different stations as and when required. Although they were paid a healthy wage, they had to work long hours for it. Homesickness was also a problem and several people's' tenure as an announcer was brief. In addition to the ones already mentioned, other staff announcers included Thorp Deveraux, Nancy Crown, Henry Cuthbertson, Graham Wilson and Hilary Wontner.

The IBC moved to bigger and better premises further up Portland Place just about 200 yards from broadcasting house. At first, the BBC seemed unconcerned by this new rival but became increasingly irritated as time passed. Firstly, there was the similar name IBC – BBC. Even the company logos and documentation were comparable in design. When the BBC started the Empire service, Plugge countered with his own IBC Empire service on short wave from EAQ Madrid.

The early style of 'live' sponsored programming, with a presenter simply linking records, was quickly replaced by more complex productions as radio expanded. Some of the output was imported from across the Atlantic. U.S.A favourites such as Stella Dallas, Backstage Wife and Young Widow Jones were regularly heard on Radio Normandy.

Nevertheless, nearly all sponsored shows on the Continental stations were pre-recorded in Britain. As mentioned earlier, these shows were mostly recorded on gramophone records. However the fragility of these discs meant a more robust style of recording was sought. IBC's connection to Gaumont British Cinemas provided the perfect solution. Sponsored shows were recorded on to the soundtrack of film reels and played back using projection equipment.

The production of sponsored shows meant that advertising agencies had to adapt the way they operated and became programme makers as well. However agencies with only a few select clients couldn't economically establish their own production facilities so IBC quickly stepped in and offered its services for hire. The Universal Programmes Corporation, as the new division became known, produced over 2000 programmes in the first three years of its existence.

Other advertising agencies involved in programme making included the London Press Exchange and the J. Walter Thompson Organisation. The London Press Exchange, produced programmes at the HMV recording studio at Abbey Road. Over at Bush House in the Strand, J. Walter Thompson introduced the Philips-Miller system of recording sound on metal tape. The investment was immense but continuous recording on tape swiftly showed financial returns.

Not all radio advertising took the form of sponsored programmes. For example, Ingersoll watches sponsored the time signal on Radio Normandy. There were also a certain number of 'spots' sold, which were usually read live by studio announcers. These scripts were read out at suitable intervals between programmes.

The scripts for Renis Face Cream were far more elaborate than the usual style. They utilised a storytelling format to capture the imagination of the listener. A romantic story was concocted about archaeologists unearthing a long-forgotten formula for beauty cream. The story progressed gradually over time and listeners would hear the latest instalment each time they tuned in.

Like the BBC in its early days, The IBC encountered a great degree of suspicion from the British Press. The Newspaper Proprietors Association regarded these stations as a deadly threat to their own advertising revenues and refused to publicise them.

One exception to this ban was the Sunday Referee, a highly regarded sporting paper that had became a family Sunday paper. Valentine Smith ran the newspaper. He had been the Circulation and Publicity Director of the Daily Mail. It was Smith's idea to introduce the 'Radio Yacht" to boost circulation of his newspaper. He realised how successful this had been and decided to involve the Sunday Referee in broadcasting if he could. It ran several broadcasts on the European Stations and regularly featured programme details within its pages. This was cited as one of the main reasons why it trebled its circulation figures.

The Newspaper Proprietors Association denied the Sunday Referee access to its transport and distribution infrastructure. Country-wide distribution was too big an undertaking for a single paper of the Referee's size to embark upon unaided. Eventually the Sunday Referee was forced to withdraw from radio altogether.

As the IBC stations were unable to get their programme details published in the newspapers they launched their own listings magazine. 'Radio Pictorial - the all-family radio paper', was launched in 1934. This publication was a lot less formal than its stuffy BBC equivalent – The Radio Times. Radio Pictorial contained pictures of radio personalities and gossipy articles about the programmes. It was the 1930s equivalent of the glossy showbiz magazines of today.

Perhaps the Newspaper Proprietors Association's aggressive tactics towards the IBC and its supporters was encouraged at a higher level. The British government were openly hostile towards the continental stations. They persuaded royalty organisations to overcharge them for permission to play recorded material and encouraged the BBC to boycott any artist or presenter who had worked on a continental station. It would seem that the government were anxious to suppress any means of mass communication over which they had no control. In 1936 a committee looking at all aspects of radio stated, 'Foreign commercial broadcasting should be discouraged by every available means.'

Radio Normandy remained the flagship station of the IBC. A new studio building and improved transmitter site was required so building work began at Louvetot (20km to the south of Fécamp) in November 1935. The new transmitter site took just over three years to complete. Broadcasts from the new studios at Caudebec began on December 12th 1938 and the new premises were officially opened on June 4th 1939. However the new studio and transmitter fell silent on September 7th at the outbreak of Word War II.

Plugge's IBC successfully demonstrated that state monopolies such as the BBC could be broken. Other parties became attracted to the idea of creating a new commercial radio station specifically for this purpose.

Once of these organisations was a French company called Radio Publicity Limited. The Company Chairman M. Jacques Gonat was a man of considerable influence in France. He hired time on Radio Paris and looked for advertisers in Britain.

Radio Paris was already established and very well equipped, with a power fifteen times greater than that of Radio Normandy. The first programme was broadcast on Sunday 29th November 1931 with Rex Palmer, an ex BBC man, at the microphone. Palmer introduced 'A Concert of HMV Records'.

However Gonat's enterprise became a victim of its own success. Radio Paris attracted so many British advertisers that it incurred the wrath of French listeners. Hearing the English language so frequently on their number-one station irritated them. The French Government interceded and forced the English Service to leave.

In 1924, Francois Aneu built a 100-watt transmitter in the Grand Duchy of Luxembourg. Because Luxembourg is centrally located in Western Europe, it was ideally placed to reach audiences in many nations, including the United Kingdom. On May 11th 1929 he brought together a group of mainly French entrepreneurs and formed the Luxembourg Society for Radio Studies as a pressure group to force the Luxembourg government to issue them a commercial broadcasting licence.

On December 19th 1929, the Luxembourg Government passed a law that would allow one company to operate a commercial radio broadcasting franchise from the Grand Duchy. Ten days later the licence was awarded to the Society, which formed the Luxembourg Broadcasting Company. The new station would be identified on the air as Radio Luxembourg.

In May 1932, Radio Luxembourg began test transmissions directed at Britain and Ireland. This provoked a hostile reaction from the

British Government. The long wave band used for these tests produced a much better signal than anything previously received from outside the country. The British Government accused Radio Luxembourg of 'pirating' the various wavelengths it was testing. The station had planned to commence regular broadcasts on June 4th 1933 but the complaints caused Radio Luxembourg to keep shifting its wavelength.

On January 1st 1934, a new international agreement, the 'European Wavelength Plan, came into effect. The Luxembourg Government refused to sign this agreement and shortly afterwards Radio Luxembourg started a regular schedule of English-language radio transmissions. The broadcasts used a new 200 kW transmitter on 1304 metres (230 kHz) in the long wave band. It quickly became such a significant part of the broadcasting fabric and millions favoured it's laid back style to the more formal approach of the BBC.

The English service was leased to Radio Publicity (London) Ltd. Luxembourg's first English transmission was fixed as December 3rd 1933. This was to coincide with the last transmission from Radio Paris. So on that occasion the two stations broadcast the same output simultaneously. Frequent announcements were made stating that all future broadcasts would emanate from Luxembourg only. Listeners were invited to retune from Paris to Luxembourg and mark the new position on the dial.

Stephen Williams was appointed as the first manager of the English language service. He arrived in Luxembourg with several hundred records and a couple of hampers of musical arrangements. Although only in his twenties, Stephen Williams was already a radio veteran. In 1928, he had secured a job as the announcer on the 'broadcasting yacht' sponsored by the Daily Mail. Prior to his appointment at Luxembourg, Williams had been Director of English Programmes at Radio Paris and had also worked briefly at Radio Normandy. Williams resumed his duties at Radio Luxembourg when the station restarted after the war. He left Luxembourg in 1948 and worked as a freelance broadcaster until 1975.

He returned to the station one last time on December 30th 1991 when Radio Luxembourg's English service closed down its medium wave service on 208 metres. The 83-year-old veteran made the final announcement, "Good luck, good listening ... and goodbye".

In the years up to the Second World War Radio Luxembourg gained a large audience in the UK and other European countries with sponsored programming aired from noon until midnight on Sundays and at various times during the rest of the week.

One of Radio Luxembourg's great successes during this period was a show aimed at children. Ovaltine, the manufacturers of a hot chocolate malt drink, first sponsored 'The Ovaltineys' in 1935. The show, broadcast on Sunday evenings between 5.30pm and 6pm, was an immediate and massive success. The club associated with the show had attracted 5 million members by 1939. Members of the club received a membership badge and book and the chance to take part in competitions and other activities. There was a weekly comic too. The programme's theme song is permanently ingrained on many generations of British people's memories.

We are the Ovaltineys,
Little girls and boys;
Make your requests, we'll not refuse you,
We are here just to amuse you.
Would you like a song or story,
Will you share our joys?
At games and sports we're more than keen;
No merrier children could be seen,
Because we all drink Ovaltine,
We're happy girls and boys!

Radio Lyons was the last of the Continental stations to broadcast English programmes in December 1936. Tony Melrose was the first announcer. Radio Lyons were keen to promote Melrose as a romantic figure and personality rather than just an announcer. In a series of magazine articles he was billed as 'the golden voice of Radio Lyons'.

Radio Lyons also heavily promoted another personality. Photographs of 'The Mystery Man of Radio Lyons' were distributed to magazines. These photographs featured a masked figure along with details of the programme he presented. The Mystery Man's show 'Film Time' was broadcast daily and sponsored by Campbell's soups.

The other output was the usual sponsored programmes and featured acts such as Carson Robinson and his Oxydol Pioneers and Carrol

Gibbons under various pseudonyms. The advertisers included Stork Margarine, Dolcis Shoes Zam-Buk, Bile Beans and Drene Shampoo. The H. Samuel Everite Time Signal was played out between the programmes. These transmissions were arranged by Broadcast Advertising Limited of London and produced by Vox Productions of Soho.

In the early hours of September 1st 1939, German forces invaded Poland. The world was about to be plunged into conflict and the network of European stations broadcasting to Britain faced an uncertain future. Some stations realised it would be impossible for private companies to continue and closed down immediately. Others vainly attempted to carry on until events, or the Nazis, overtook them.

There followed a period of consolidation as each European country's radio stations were gradually brought under governmental control. During the war radio would become a powerful aide in the dissemination of information and propaganda. In addition to the physical conflict, a war of words was about to be waged for the hearts and minds of radio listeners around the world.

7

Radio at War

With Hitler's invasion of Poland on September 1st 1939, the British Prime Minister Neville Chamberlain's policy of appeasement had failed. On that day, the Regional Programme was suddenly discontinued and merged with the National to become the Home Service. This attenuated service continued for the first six months of the war.

The BBC had been preparing for the outbreak of the Second World War for some months. All Home Service transmissions were transmitted on two frequencies (668 kHz and 767 kHz) with the network of transmitters synchronised together to obstruct direction-finding capabilities. It was feared that the transmitters might have been used as a navigational aid by enemy aircraft. The television service was also suspended for the same reason. The number of television receivers in the London reception area had risen to 23,000 by this time.

On the morning of Sunday 3rd September 1939, Prime Minister Neville Chamberlain announced that Britain was at war with Germany. The speech was relayed direct from the cabinet room at 10 Downing Street. King George VI's message to Britain and the Empire was broadcast that evening.

On the day Britain declared war, listening to the BBC was made illegal in Germany. The Nazis had been jamming BBC broadcasts experimentally for several months prior to the start of hostilities. After September 3rd 1939 the jamming increased. The BBC retaliated by increasing transmitter power and adding extra frequencies. Later, leaflets were dropped over cities in occupied Europe. The leaflets contained instructions detailing how to construct a directional loop aerial that would enable listeners to hear the stations through the jamming.

The BBC Home Service mainly concentrated on news and informational programmes in the early days of the war. There were now ten news broadcasts daily. There had been five before war broke out. Nearly half the nation listened to the 9 o'clock news each evening. This was because of the nightly war reports from distinguished correspondents such as Richard Dimbleby, Frank Gillard, Godfrey Talbot and Wynford Vaughan-Thomas.

In the first couple of months these reports included an eyewitness account from Edinburgh of the German air raid on the Firth of Forth, Richard Dimbleby reporting from the British Expeditionary Force's headquarters in France and an interview with survivors of the Athenia, the British liner torpedoed by the Germans.

In addition there were frequent pep talks given by Ministers and civil servants. Winston Churchill, First Lord of the Admiralty, made his first wartime broadcast on October 1st 1939. These talks and news bulletins were punctuated by countless gramophone records. A new programme called 'The Home Front' started on the 30th September. This programme detailed aspects of wartime life in Britain.

Sandy MacPherson the organist was gainfully employed during the first fortnight of the war. MacPherson played up to twelve hours per day, also filling in with announcements and programme notes whilst the organisation hastily evacuated its staff from London to various locations around the British Isles. His normal signature tune was 'Happy Days Are Here Again' but this would have been highly inappropriate so it was swiftly replaced by one of his own compositions.

The outbreak of war immediately affected staff numbers at the corporation. A lot of BBC staff were reservists and went off to serve in the forces. In addition, each post was graded and only essential personnel were kept on. The rest were told to find alternative employment for the duration.

Although they weren't directly involved at this point, the American public were continuously being informed of the worsening situation in Europe. American journalists had been constantly reporting back home as Europe was mobilizing for war. Hans von (H. V.) Kaltenborn became renowned for his broadcasts from Europe, where he conversed with world leaders such as Mussolini and Adolf Hitler. His broadcasts from Spain during the civil war helped to rally American opinion against fascism. Kaltenborn attended when British Prime Minister Neville Chamberlain flew to Germany to meet Hitler. Kaltenborn translated and interpreted events for the American public. The Munich crisis made him the nation's leading broadcast journalist.

Edward R. Murrow, another CBS reporter managed to broadcast from Vienna during the annexation of Austria and went on to make gripping reports from London during the Blitz. The American correspondents reported on the distribution of gas masks in Prague, Hitler's fiery threats from Berlin and the paralysis of the French cabinet in Paris.

Radio Luxembourg's English service closed down on September 1st 1939. This was because the Luxembourg Government wanted to avoid any accusations of bias. The Luxembourg government adopted a careful non-belligerent stance towards its neighbours in order to prevent a German invasion. The last thing broadcast was a march written by a local composer called 'For Liberty'. The Germans occupied Luxembourg in May 1940 and incorporated the station's facilities into the German network.

Most of the International Broadcasting Company stations closed down as it became obvious that war was inevitable. Radio Normandy had opened a transmitter and studio at Caudebec a few months before World War II began. The new site was immediately mothballed and wasn't used again until the German's used the facilities to broadcast propaganda to Britain. This didn't last long as the RAF bombed the transmitter out of action.

Radio Normandy's transmitter at Fécamp was used to transmit programmes from Radio International. This station's output was aimed at troops in France and the South of England during the period now known as the 'phoney war'. It broadcast for thirteen hours a day and featured old IBC programmes with the sponsored messages removed. On Christmas Day 1939, special shows featuring stars like Charlie Kunz, Tessie O'Shea and George Formby were transmitted.

Radio International even published its own magazine 'Happy Listening', which was distributed free to all active units of the British forces. The name of the magazine was a direct link to Radio Normandy as the station had used the slogan 'Happy Listening' in their programme listings in Radio Pictorial. Only two issues were published as the station had a relatively short lifespan. Radio International lasted until January 3rd 1940. It's thought that pressure from the French and British Governments forced the closure.

During the war the BBC's transmission equipment was placed under the direction of Fighter Command. The old Daventry 5XX long wave transmitter was converted to medium wave operation and joined the Home Service network. The 150kW Droitwich long wave transmitter was also converted to medium wave operation and, together with the other former National Programme transmitters, was synchronised on 1149 kHz and broadcast the European Service at night.

At a later date the Start Point transmitter in South East Devon was converted for use on 1149 kHz and together with Droitwich these two transmitters broadcast the European Service, leaving other transmitters available for a new third service to be added later.

The synchronisation of the Home Service transmitters on to just two frequencies caused numerous interference problems for domestic listeners, with one Home Service transmitter interfering with another on the same frequency. To surmount this problem the BBC installed a group of 61 low power relay stations around the UK using 203 metres (1474 kHz) called 'Group H', and which was later extended. This network of low power relays filled in the coverage gaps from the main transmitters. All of the Group H stations were manned 24 hours per day so the broadcasts could be terminated at a moment's notice if air raid conditions warranted it.

In September 1941, the 5XX transmitter at Daventry, the Droitwich transmitter and a new transmitter installed at Brookman's Park were established as a long wave network of transmitters to broadcast the European Service on 200 kHz. A high power transmitter at Ottringham in the East Yorkshire Riding was added in February 1943, also using 200 kHz. The Ottringham transmitting station was a massive installation consisting of six 500 feet high masts and 800 kilowatt transmitters.

The BBC deployed a lot of staff to other areas of the United Kingdom to avoid frequent bombing raids. However this was not a foolproof plan as several BBC installations also came under attack. On 19th November 1940, the Adderley Park transmitter in Birmingham was totally destroyed and several staff sheltering nearby were killed. The BBC premises in Swansea were totally destroyed in February 1941.

The BBC staff members that remained in London were extremely vulnerable to attack as the German 'Blitzkrieg' intensified. In October 1940, a delayed-action bomb killed seven people, injured many others and blew out part of the west side of Broadcasting House. Listeners to the nine o'clock news heard the announcer pause, and then continue.

In December 1940, a land mine caused so much damage to Broadcasting House that the European service had to be moved temporarily to Maida Vale. The following April all premises on the eastern half of the Broadcasting House site were totally destroyed by high-explosive bombs. A month later, Queen's Hall was demolished during a raid and the Maida Vale studios suffered a direct hit by a high-explosive bomb.

The BBC's European service had decamped temporarily to Maida Vale but eventually a new home was found. This was Bush House, where there were already some basement studios and offices. This had previously been the production home of Advertising Agency J. Walter Thomson during the 1930s. Bush House also suffered bomb damage from a flying bomb in June 1944. The statue representing America lost its left arm and was restored in 1977.

Bush House stands between Australia House and India House on the semi-circular island of buildings called Aldwych, in Westminster, London. Designed by Harvey Corbett, Bush House was built in 1923 and opened in 1925. Further wings were added between 1928 and 1935.

This quintessentially British building was originally constructed by an Anglo-American trading organisation headed by Irving T. Bush. This is who the building its named after. At the time it was built it was declared the 'most expensive building in the world', having cost around £2 million.

All of the BBC's foreign language services gradually invaded Bush House, permeating each wing in turn. It was the home of the BBC World Service for seven decades. However the BBC's lease expired in 2012 and all world service staff transferred to Broadcasting House.

Although the BBC retained a degree of independence the organisation had to adhere to Ministry of Information 'guidance'. This censorship took two forms. One covered the morale of the nation and the other protected defence forces' security. Any script had to have the two official stamps before it was broadcast. The locations of troops, cabinet members or the Royal Family were never given. Weather forecasts were banned, as this would reveal suitable conditions for bombing.

The seeming failure of the British government, including the military failure in Norway in 1940, meant that criticism of Neville Chamberlain became more and more forceful. Chamberlain stood down and Winston Churchill became Prime Minister on May 10th 1940. He swiftly emerged to be the most dominant figure in British politics during the war. For many people, Churchill's stand summarised why the war was being fought.

His radio speeches are often credited with helping the Allied forces to win the war. However rumours later emerged that a stand-in had delivered many of his radio speeches, as he was too busy elsewhere. This had always been denied by official sources but a BBC 78rpm record was later unearthed to back up the story. Shortly before his death in 1980, the actor Norman Shelley revealed that he had been the substitute for Churchill. To confuse matters further, Churchill agreed to record some of his most memorable lines for the BBC after the war. It's these speeches that are retained in the official BBC archives.

The BBC Home Service had been implemented in a hurry and many of the pre-war favourite programmes had been dropped. For a while the Home Service broadcast a mixture of programmes but eventually the news programmes remained on the Home Service while the music and light entertainment shows transferred to a new service.

During the period known as the 'Phoney War' it became clear that members of the armed services were now mainly sat in barracks with little to do. The BBC Forces Programme was launched on Sunday 7th January 1940 to appeal directly to these men.

Its mixture of drama, comedy, popular music, features, quiz shows and variety was richer and more varied than the former National Programme. Although intended for soldiers the Forces Programme was also a hit with large numbers of British civilians.

Programmes such as 'Danger - Men at Work' and "Hi Gang" were aimed at the forces generally. However other shows were also developed for specific services including "Garrison Theatre" for the

Army and "Ack Ack Beer Beer" for the anti-aircraft and barrage balloon stations.

The people working on the Home Front were not forgotten either. Music While You Work was a music programme broadcast twice daily to British factory workers on the BBC General Forces Programme. It began on Sunday June 23rd 1940 following a Government proposal that daily broadcasts of cheerful music piped into the factories would improve morale and increase production. The first programme featured Dudley Beaven at the theatre organ with the afternoon edition's music provided by a trio called The Organolists.

The organs were phased out gradually as it was felt their tone was incompatible with factory conditions. Small instrumental ensembles ballroom dance orchestras, light orchestras, brass and military bands replaced them as they were considered to be more suitable. Nevertheless not every instrument was welcome on the show. Pizzicato violin playing proved to be inaudible due to background noise in the factories. Drummers were banned from playing 'rim shots' as these apparently sounded like gunfire over factory tannoy systems.

Initially, the programme had no signature tune, but light music composer Eric Coates had written a melody called 'Calling All Workers' and this was adopted as the signature tune from October 1940. A third edition of the show was introduced at 10.30pm for night-shift workers. By the end of the war 5 million workers in over 9000 factories were tuning in. The programme continued after the war and remained a regular broadcasting fixture until 1967.

Worker's Playtime was another programme designed to boost the nation's morale. Broadcast from factory canteens around Britain, it was one of the first touring variety shows on the BBC. Many well-known acts were given their first break on the show including Peter Sellers, Tony Hancock, Frankie Howerd, Ann Shelton, Julie Andrews, Morecambe and Wise, Ken Dodd and Bob Monkhouse. The show made its debut on May 31st 1941, originally scheduled to run for six weeks it continued until 1964. Bill Gates was the producer for the entire 23 years that the show was on air. Gates would end each programme with the words 'Good Luck All Workers'.

Popular American variety programming was imported for the first time – "The Charlie MacCarthy Show", "The Bob Hope Show" and "The Jack Benny Hour" were all heard on the Forces Programme. Vera Lynn's programme 'Sincerely Yours' was a big hit with the listeners and she swiftly became the 'Forces Sweetheart'. However the programme was less popular with the BBC Board of Governors. The minutes of one meeting dismissed the programme with the words "Popularity noted, but deplored".

The most popular British comedy programme during the war years was ITMA starring Tommy Handley, a well-known Liverpudlian comedian. Handley was a veteran radio performer whose debut broadcast was a relay of the Royal Command Performance of December 1923. The show's name was an acronym of a topical catchphrase of the time. In the run up to the war, whenever Hitler made some new territorial claim, the newspaper headlines would proclaim 'It's That Man Again'.

The programme began on July 12th 1939 with a series of four fortnightly shows. The first episodes were based onboard a pirate commercial radio ship. However these initial shows received a lukewarm response and a new format was quickly sought. In the early days of the war, new Government Ministries sprang up overnight. So for the second series Tommy Handley became Minister of Aggravation and Mysteries at the Office of Twerps.

ITMA returned on 19th September 1939 for a weekly series of 21 episodes. These were transmitted from Bristol, where the BBC Variety Department had moved, hoping to avoid the heavy bombing raids directed at London.

Handley was the only survivor from the original series and a brand new supporting cast was assembled. These included Vera Lennox as Handley's secretary Dotty and Maurice Denham as Mrs. Tickle the office cleaner. Sam Costa and Jack Train provided other characters including Funf, the elusive German spy. The catchphrase 'this is Funf speaking' found its way into many private telephone calls over the next few years. This series proved very popular and the show was swiftly re-commissioned.

Before the third series started the BBC Variety Department had moved yet again to Bangor in North Wales. The war situation was deteriorating and it was thought that spoofs of Government

Departments would not be acceptable. The show began a six week summer season on June 20th 1941 and was renamed 'It's That Sand Again' It was set in a sleepy seaside resort called Foaming at the Mouth. In the new series Tommy Handley became the town's Mayor.

There was another change of cast with only Jack Train returning. In came Sydney Keith, Horace Percival, Dorothy Summers and Fred Yule. Several famous characters were launched during this short run. These included Lefty and Sam the gangsters and Deepend Dan the Diver. Other popular characters included Claude and Cecil the over polite handymen and Ali Oop, a shady Middle Eastern hawker.

The show reverted to its original name for the fourth series and the popular seaside setting was retained. In this series the team were joined by Dino Galvani as Tommy Handley's Italian secretary Signor So-So and Clarence Wright as a hapless commercial traveller who never made a sale. Dorothy Summers introduced the famous office cleaner, Mrs. Mopp. Her catchphrase 'Can I do yer now sir?' became immensely popular.

The next three series of ITMA continued in the same vein apart from a few minor cast changes. During this period a film version of the show was produced and was received warmly. The cast were also invited to perform a special show at Windsor Castle to celebrate Princess Elizabeth's 16th birthday. One of the newer characters to appear during this period was Colonel Humphrey Chinstrap. The colonel would turn almost any innocent remark into the offer of a drink with his catchphrase 'I don't mind if I do'.

ITMA returned for its seventh series in October 1943 with another revamp. Handley was now Squire of Much Fiddling. Over the next year several special editions were recorded at various military bases. These included the Navy base at Scapa Flow and a garrison theatre 'somewhere in England'.

The show was immensely popular with nearly 40% of the population listening at times. ITMA continued after the war but the series ended abruptly after the scheduled broadcast on January 6th 1949. Tommy Handley passed away three days later and the BBC wisely decided to let the show die with him.

The war had forced a change to the BBC's pre-war policy of broadcasting only serious or religious programmes on the Sabbath.

Looking at the programme listings for May 1941 showed that over three hours of light entertainment shows were broadcast on Sunday evenings. There would be no reverting back to Reith's Sunday policy after the war.

The BBC commenced its "V for Victory" campaign at midnight on July 20th 1941. The "V for Victory" broadcasts started with a message from Prime Minister Winston Churchill aimed at the European countries under occupation by the Nazis. "The V sign is the symbol of the unconquerable will of the people of the occupied territories and a portent of the fate awaiting the Nazi tyranny." From that point on the BBC's broadcasts used a call sign that utilised the opening bars of Beethoven's 5th Symphony, which has the same rhythm as the Morse code for the letter V (dot-dot-dot-dash).

When the American servicemen arrived en masse in 1943 and 1944 in preparation for Operation Overlord, they found even the livelier Forces Programme shows to be staid and slow compared with the existing output of the American networks.

On July 4th 1943, the American Forces Network (AFN) was introduced on 344 metres. Using BBC emergency facilities at 11 Carlos Place in London, the signal was fed by landline to five regional transmitters. The initial broadcasts included less than five hours of recorded shows, a BBC newscast and a sportscast.

AFN provided a morale-boosting service of record programmes that was popular with the American forces. However AFN was equally popular with British audiences, who could hear records and music not usually heard on the BBC.

During the next 11 months, the daily broadcasts expanded to 19 hours. 50 additional transmitters were installed (Including six in Northern Ireland). Six additional staff joined the original complement of seven broadcasters and technicians.

It was the popularity of AFN and the increasing numbers of American forces based in Britain that persuaded the BBC to 'fine tune' their Forces Programme. Finally in response to a direct appeal from General Eisenhower, the BBC abolished the Forces Programme and established the General Forces Programme on February 27th 1944.

The new service's output was lighter and less formal than its predecessor with material that would be popular with the American and Canadian troops. The station assumed a more North American style and played more American material. American shows like 'The Bob Hope Show' 'Amos and Andy' and 'Command Performance' were broadcast.

They soon found that this new approach was a big hit with everyone, not just the troops, and certainly helped the listeners endure this troubled period. Regulars such as Canadian Announcer Charmian Sansom, Joan Dallas and the Robert Farnon Canadian Army Band became firm favourites.

AFN London moved from its original BBC studios to 80 Portland Place in May 1944. As D-Day approached, AFN combined with the BBC and the Canadian Broadcasting Corporation to form the Allied Expeditionary Forces Programme. The AEF programme made its debut on 285 metres at 0600 on June 6th 1944. The signature tune 'Oranges and Lemons', was followed by the opening announcement from Margaret Hubble. The first show was a record programme called 'Rise and Shine'. U.S Seargeant Dick Dudley and AC2 Ronnie Waldman co-hosted the show.

AFN and BBC personnel accompanied the invasion force when allied troops landed in France. They sent news reports back to studio locations in London. In addition AFN set up a network of mobile stations to broadcast music and news to the troops in the field.

As allied troops advanced through Europe. AFN mobile stations were set up at Paris, Nice, Marseilles, Rheims, Le Havre, Cannes and Biarritz. AFN's administrative headquarters remained in London but its operational headquarters moved to Paris. When Germany surrendered on May 8th 1945, the network had grown to some 700 people and 63 stations scattered throughout Central Europe.

There was another radio service backed by the Americans. The American Broadcasting Station in Europe (ABSIE) began on April 30th 1944, five weeks before D-Day. It was established by the Office of War Information (OWI) and the Supreme Headquarters Allied Expeditionary Force's (SHAEF) Psychological Warfare Division. ABSIE broadcast from underground studios in Wardour Street in the London district of Soho. The station's brief was to provide "the truth of this war to our friends in Europe - and to our enemies". Colonel William Paley, peacetime head of CBS, was drafted in to run the operation. He negotiated with the BBC for equipment and pledged that ABSIE would disband 90 days after V - E Day.

The station provided news and information in seven languages. There was a news bulletin presented at dictation speed for use by the underground press in occupied countries. It also featured talks by exiled leaders as King Haakon of Norway and Jan Masaryk of Czechoslovakia.

Not surprisingly ABSIE's most popular programmes were music shows. According to captured Germans, the favourite Allied programme heard in Germany was Music for the Wehrmacht. This show featured top American acts like Dinah Shore, Glen Miller and Bing Crosby introducing their songs by reading from phonetic German scripts. The American Broadcasting Station in Europe only lasted for fourteen months. Colonel Paley fulfilled his promise to the BBC and closed the station shortly after V - E Day.

The BBC's German Service had continued to broadcast throughout the war and by 1942 the German service was broadcasting around six hours per day. They had employed a policy of restraint in the early years of the war and took great pains to maintain a level of neutrality. This approach began to pay dividends and audience levels steadily rose.

The German Service adopted a relaxed and calm tone for its broadcasts. This broadcasting style was more akin to pre-war Radio Luxembourg than the BBC Home Service. The announcers relaxed manner contrasted sharply with the frenetic style of the Nazi broadcasts.

The most listened to programme on the BBC's German service was transmitted every afternoon. 'Aus der Freien Welt' (From the Free World) introduced by Spike Hughes. He played hot jazz and swing records that were banned in Germany. The records were interspersed by news and short talks.

The German service also featured monologues and sketches. One of the more popular series featured a character called Adolf Hirnschal, a German private, writing letters home to his wife. An Austrian refugee actor and writer called Robert Ehrenzweig, who became known as Robert Lucas in Britain, wrote the scripts for these monologues. Other popular radio characters on the German Service included 'Blockleiter Braunmüller' (Blockleader Brownmiller) and 'Frau Wernicke' (Mrs Wernicke). Bruno Adler, another German writer in exile, created these radio spoofs.

Clandestine stations regularly appear during periods of war or civil unrest. These stations broadcast on behalf of various governments or political movements, including rebel or insurrectionist forces. Clandestine broadcasts may emanate from transmitters located in rebel-controlled territory. Or from outside the country entirely, using another country's transmission facilities.

Radio can be a highly effective propaganda tool and both sides utilised it extensively during the war. There are essentially three different types of propaganda – white, grey and black. White is the most common type of propaganda where the real source is declared. Usually more accurate information is given, if also slanted or distorted. With grey propaganda, the source is never identified. Black propaganda is false information and material that claims to be from a source on one side of a conflict, but is really from the opposing side. It is typically used to vilify, humiliate or misrepresent the enemy. These black propaganda radio stations often pretended to broadcast illegally from within the countries they targeted.

The British Government launched several black propaganda stations during World War Two. These operations were the responsibility of the Political Warfare Executive based near Woburn Abbey. This unit produced black propaganda radio stations in most of the languages of occupied Europe.

Amongst the various language services, two were aimed at Italy. These were Radio Italy and Radio Liberty, which revealed curious intimate details of Mussolini's private life. The Italian stations were suspended when it quickly became apparent that the Italian farmers and workers didn't have short wave radios and therefore couldn't receive the broadcasts.

Not surprisingly most of these clandestine stations broadcast in the German language. The mastermind behind this unit was Sefton Delmer, who had been the Berlin correspondent of the Daily Express prior to the outbreak of the war. He was able to speak German perfectly and had specialist knowledge of the Nazis. He had met most of the top party members, including Hitler, during his time in Berlin.

Selmer's first effort was a right wing short wave station called Gustav Siegfried Eins (George Sugar One). To front this station they invented a character called Der Chef (The Chief). This individual professed to be a Nazi extremist who accused Hitler and his henchmen of going soft. The station focused on alleged corruption and included salacious stories regarding the sexual proclivities of Hitler Youth Leaders. There were also frequent stories concerning the outrageous sexual behaviour of Nazi party bosses with the wives of absent Wehrmacht troops.

Selmer and the Political Warfare Executive created a grey propaganda station for the Navy. This was the station Atlantiksender, broadcasting non-stop music and news for the u-boat crews. Although most of the U-boat crews realised that Atlantiksender had allied origins they became genuinely troubled at just how much the enemy knew. With a growing first-rate intelligence department, daily intelligence reports from the Navy and the Combined Services they gained valuable details to add to their stories.

These stations were designed to demoralise and spread dissension amongst the German troops. Information for these stations was gathered from various sources such as secret service reports, censorship intercepts, newspaper items and RAF reconnaissance reports. They also used information and names of actual people gleaned from captured German sailors, soldiers, and airmen. Actual news was interspersed with fake items. One false report revealed that tests had shown that a large quantity of blood used in German army field hospitals was contaminated with syphilis.

On November 8th 1942, the British installed a high power medium wave broadcasting transmitter near Crowborough in the Ashdown Forest in Sussex. It was nicknamed Aspidistra after the Gracie Fields song 'The Biggest Aspidistra in the World'. Aspidistra could switch frequencies and wave bands almost instantly and was used extensively for propaganda broadcasts.

Despite its strategic importance, the Crowborough transmitter never suffered a direct attack by German aircraft. On one occasion, an aircraft offloaded its cargo of incendiary devices a mile from the site.

However this was thought to have been a standard raid and Aspidistra was not the main target. There was another incident when a V1 rocket skimmed over the hill at Crowborough, which was the highest point before London. The doodlebug flew under the guy-wires of the mast and continued on its way to the capital.

Selmer's next project was a 24 hour broadcasting station on medium wave. Soldatensender Calais (Calais Armed Forces Radio) was introduced just a few weeks before the invasion of France. Soldatensender brought the first news of the D Day landings to the world. The communication breakdown between German units at this point was so severe that many commanders tuned in to the station for situation reports. They would use these reports to correct the constantly changing battle plans on their staff maps. This information was correct 99 times out of a 100. However on the hundredth it would drive the Germans into a trap set by the allies.

The attempted assassination of Hitler was exactly what the Woburn Abbey team had been waiting for. They maximised the opportunity by implicating as many as possible in the plot. Emboldened by this development, the Soldatensender demanded that an end be put to the war to save Germany.

As the allied forces advanced across Europe, Radio Luxembourg and the BBC were telling the German civilians to 'stay put'. Winston Churchill was outraged by this and instructed the Black Propagandists to try to unsettle the German people and cause as much disruption as they possibly could.

Soldatensender broadcast a bogus report saying that seven bomb-free zones had been established in Central and South Germany. It stated that these areas would be supervised by neutral Red Cross representatives and refugees would be safe from further enemy air attacks. Sending the civilians on to the roads of Germany would disrupt supplies and block the German army's retreat.

Also with first class intelligence information and using advanced knowledge of Allied air raids, Delmer's team were able to predict which station would go off the air and when. As the German station went silent they would take over the German network. Specially trained announcers would make bogus announcements identical in rhythm and tone of the genuine station.

The Nazis also realised the potential of propaganda broadcasts. "Germany Calling" was broadcast to audiences in Great Britain on the medium wave station Reichssender Hamburg and by short wave to the United States of America. Radio Luxembourg's transmitters were also used to relay the broadcasts.

Germany's propaganda broadcasts stemmed mainly from Berlin but to prevent their transmissions from being bombed out the Nazis had perfected an ingenious network of mobile transmitters. An extensive system of landlines was located along all the major routes in Germany. Every few kilometres there was a concrete box where engineers could plug in their equipment. Mobile broadcasting units stored in the back of trucks were moved around like chess pieces to these connection points. They would stay there for a few hours and move on before the allied bombers could pinpoint their location.

The Reich Ministry of Public Enlightenment and Propaganda was led by Dr Joseph Goebbels, a master propagandist. The Nazi transmissions gave prominence to reports on the sinking of ships and the shooting down of aircraft. German radio frequently rang a mock lutine bell to announce the sinking of a British vessel.

Although the broadcasts were widely known to be Nazi propaganda, Allied troops and civilians frequently listened to these broadcasts. Despite the inaccuracies and exaggerations, they frequently offered the only details available from behind enemy lines concerning the fate of friends and relatives who did not return from bombing raids over Germany.

The most prominent Nazi propaganda broadcaster was William Joyce. Nicknamed Lord Haw-Haw by British listeners, Joyce was Irish by blood, American by birth and carried a British passport. Joyce had been interested in politics from an early age. Both he and his father, rather unusually for Irish Catholics at the time, were both Unionists and openly supported British rule.

In 1924, after attending a Conservative Party meeting at the Lambeth Baths in Battersea, Joyce was accosted by a gang and subjected to a vicious attack. He received a deep razor cut that sliced across his right cheek from behind the earlobe all the way to the corner of his mouth. After spending two weeks in hospital he was left with a disfiguring facial scar. Joyce was convinced that his attackers were 'Jewish communists' and the incident became a major influence on the rest of his life.

He joined the British Union of Fascists in 1932 and fled to Germany just before the war broke out in 1939. Joyce had been tipped off that the British authorities intended to detain him as a Nazi sympathiser. On arrival, he immediately became a broadcaster for Joseph Goebbels' Propaganda Ministry and broadcast weekly from 1939 to 1945.

Many of Joyce's stories were designed to unnerve the British public. On one occasion, Joyce asked the British public to question the Admiralty over the aircraft carrier "Ark Royal". In fact, nothing had happened to the "Ark Royal" but the seeds of doubt had been sown. It is thought that on average six million people listened to Joyce each broadcast. Many found the broadcasts so absurd that they were seen as a way of relieving the tedium of life in Britain during the war. William Joyce became a figure of fun. Comedians lampooned his idiosyncratic accent. There was even a song written about him – 'Lord Haw-Haw, the humbug of Hamburg'.

The public may not have taken Joyce's broadcasts seriously but that was not the case in certain areas of officialdom. A report released in January 1940 showed that, during the previous month, 30% of the adult population had listened to the broadcasts from Hamburg. The BBC came under pressure from senior politicians and military top brass to reply to Joyce's claims. However the BBC's official reply was always the same. They thought that 'a permanent, regular refutation of German lies was not possible or desirable'.

On the night of April 30th 1945, a drunken Joyce made his last broadcast from Hamburg as British troops entered the city. With his adopted world crashing down around him, but still committed to the Nazi cause, Joyce rambled on through his farewell speech. In Berlin, Hitler was simultaneously saying good bye to his entourage in anticipation of ending his life a few hours later.

Captured by the British, Joyce stood trial for treason. The court denied his claim of American citizenship because he held a British passport. He was found guilty and hanged at Wandsworth Prison on January 3rd 1946.

Lord Haw Haw's Japanese equivalent was Tokyo Rose whose mission was to demoralise the American troops in the Pacific. She was the evil seductress who urged G I's to abandon their war against the Imperial Japanese war machine.

As a matter of fact "Tokyo Rose" did not exist. There wasn't actually a female broadcaster using that particular soubriquet on the air. There was "Nanking Nancy", "Radio Rose", "Madam Tojo" and "Orphan Ann". There were at least eight women who broadcast from Radio Tokyo, and quite possibly more. The occupying forces under MacArthur identified five women as possibly being "Tokyo Rose" within days of entering Tokyo.

The woman who was ultimately branded as "Tokyo Rose" by the American press was Iva Toguri, an American born to Japanese immigrant parents. Her family did not speak Japanese in the home, nor did they adhere to Japanese customs or eat Japanese food. She had been sent to Japan to care for an ailing relative just before the outbreak of the Pacific War. For a number of reasons she had left without proper permits and found it impossible to return to America when war was declared. She was trapped in Japan, unable to speak or read the language.

Despite pressure by the Japanese authorities, Iva Toguri refused to relinquish her American citizenship. She ended up working as a typist at Radio Tokyo. As a native English speaker it was her job to edit the scripts being prepared for broadcast. Eventually Toguri was pressurised into become one of the announcers. In wartime Japan nobody disobeyed direct orders from the army.

Iva Toguri's show was called "Zero Hour". She had a light presentation style that was hugely popular with the G I's and her show quickly became the most popular radio show in the Pacific theatre. She would introduce herself as "your favourite enemy, Orphan Ann." Her comical delivery was deliberate, and removed any perceived threat from her script. Far from being a covert disseminator of misinformation, Iva openly warned her listeners that her programme contained 'dangerous and wicked propaganda, so beware!' The results were more amusing than disheartening. Instead of lowering morale, she boosted it.

After the war Iva Toguri was arrested and tried for treason. She was sentenced to ten years in prison and stripped of her prized US citizenship. Gradually, as the anti-Japanese attitude of the post-war years began to ebb, it became clear that Iva Toguri had been treated harshly. She eventually received a Presidential pardon in 1977, and her cherished citizenship was restored.

These propaganda stations gradually disappeared as the war neared its conclusion. In Europe, as the German forces retreated and countries were repatriated, the need for these stations evaporated. The most powerful of these, Soldatensender Calais, closed down finally on April 30th 1945. No formal closure announcement was made.

Sefton Delmer advised his team at Woburn Abbey to remain tight-lipped about their work with the Political Warfare Executive. He didn't want to offer the Germans the opportunity to claim they had been beaten by under-handed means and not militarily. However it's debatable whether these propaganda broadcasts had any real impact on the outcome of the war.

On September 1st 1944, five years to the day since the English service of Radio Luxembourg closed down; the German's abandoned the facilities at the Villa Louvigny. They blew up the main control room in the basement of the building but left the transmission site intact. They only destroyed the transmission valves and had left the other equipment alone. A stock of transmission valves were later discovered at the Post Office warehouse at Diekirch.

Several days later the Allies regained control of the studio and transmitter facilities. The area around the transmitter site had been mined and a tank was destroyed as it approached. However the transmission facilities were eventually cleared of all booby traps and Radio Luxembourg was handed over to the Allies.

The SHAEF (Supreme Headquarters Allied Expeditionary Force) took over the running of the station. Programmes were stralegic in nature and aimed at the German units still active in the combat zone. Programmes in the local Luxembourg dialect were introduced in October 1944. Eventually the Luxembourg transmitter relayed programmes from the BBC and ABSIE.

The Luxembourg facilities were also used to broadcast a black propaganda station called 'Radio Twelve Twelve' run by a team of Twelfth Army personnel. Four 15-minute programmes were broadcast daily. The station purported to be a German underground station and maintained an anti-Nazi stance. Its aim was to spread disinformation and unsettle the German population. It falsely reported that tanks were in the vicinity of Ludwigshafen and Nuremberg and this caused widespread panic. Radio Twelve Twelve was in existence for only 127 days but it had succeeded in its aims.

As the war in Europe began to go the Allies way there were increasing signs that life in Britain was improving. Programmes were interrupted frequently during the autumn of 1944 to bring news of the liberation of Paris, Brussels, Luxembourg, Athens and Belgrade. The chimes of Big Ben were reinstated. News bulletins carried details of the end of fireguard and Civil Defence duties in certain areas. On December 3rd the BBC news announced that the Home Guard was to be disbanded.

At 3.00pm on May 8th 1945, a victorious Winston Churchill officially announced the end of the war with Germany. Speaking from the cabinet room at Downing Street, he reminded the nation that Japan had still to be defeated but that the people of Great Britain "May allow ourselves a brief period of rejoicing. Advance Britannia. Long live the cause of freedom! God save the King! "

That evening at 9.00pm, King George VI broadcast to the nation from Buckingham Palace. This was the last official event on V.E. Day.

The cessation of hostilities in Europe didn't mean an immediate end to the BBC's General Forces Programme. It moved to short wave and continued to transmit to areas that were still engaged in active combat. Gradually Britain began to disengage from each fighting area as civilian rule was restored The General Forces Programme was slowly replaced by the BBC General Overseas Service until complete closure on December 31st 1946.

8

The End Of The Golden Age

Following the cessation of hostilities, the BBC immediately restructured its services. The provincial regional programmes resumed but the Regional Programme itself didn't. The BBC reintroduced the six pre-war regional services, on the same transmitters and frequencies as before, retaining the wartime name BBC Home Service. So for example the Scottish regional station on Medium Wave was now called the Scottish Home Service.

This was the first part of the BBC's post-war restructuring of radio into three networks. The three complementary networks were designed not only to inform and entertain, but to educate the public as well.

The second phase was implemented on July 29th 1945. The BBC Light Programme commenced broadcasting on the long wave frequencies that had previously carried the General Forces Programme. Launch day programmes included the ubiquitous Sandy Macpherson at the organ and an afternoon performance by the Torquay Municipal Orchestra.

The long wave signal was transmitted from Droitwich in the English Midlands and gave fairly good coverage of most of the UK. Some medium wave frequencies were added later, using low-power transmitters to fill in local blank spots.

The new service was generally well received. Although some listeners regretted that the American acts they had listened to on the Forces Programme had been dropped. However several long running programmes were gradually introduced including Woman's Hour', 'Dick Barton Special Agent', 'Housewife's Choice' and 'Have A Go'.

Responding to the public's growing interest in the arts, the BBC introduced The Third Programme on September 29th 1946. Broadcast initially for six hours each evening, the Corporation defined the new service as "being for the educated rather than an educational programme." It gradually became one of the leading cultural and intellectual forces in Britain, playing a crucial role in disseminating the arts.

The Third Programme was given a unique freedom from form and routine. No news bulletins or fixed periods were allowed to interfere with the output. Plays, operas, and concerts were given in their entirety.

The Third Programme became a major patron of the arts with music filling a third of the output. The network's musical output provided a wide range of serious classical music and live concerts. Symphony concerts were aired on Thursdays and Saturdays with a concert of chamber music every Monday. Jazz music was also heavily featured. The new network also played a crucial role in the development of contemporary composers such as Benjamin Britten by commissioning new works.

Speech formed a large proportion of the Third Programme's output. Its drama productions included plays by Samuel Beckett, Henry Reed, Harold Pinter and Joe Orton. It also commissioned new plays by leading writers. Probably the most celebrated of these was 'Under Milk Wood' by Dylan Thomas.

The Third Programme was for many years the single largest source of copyright payments to poets. Young writers such as Philip Larkin, David Jones and Laura Riding received early exposure on the network. The radio talk, a staple of the early days of the BBC, also made a comeback. Nationally known intellectuals such as Isiah Berlin, Fred Hoyle and Bertrand Russell were frequently heard talking on philosophy or cosmology. There was also an interesting innovation - Radio Critics would give their opinion of the "third programme" productions.

The esoteric character of the service proved to be harmful rather than advantageous to the BBC. Although the BBC was normally exalted for its noble objective of raising cultural standards, the Third Programme's high production costs and small audience figures made the service an easy target for critics and politicians.

In fact the Third Programmes existence went against the principles of its founding father. John Reith had been opposed to fragmenting audiences by splitting programming genres across different networks. From the outset though, it had influential supporters: the

Education Secretary in the Attlee government, Ellen Wilkinson, spoke rather optimistically of creating a "third programme nation".

Despite its influential supporters, and following an internal reorganisation, the cultural programmes were reduced in hours in 1957. The Third programme had to share its frequency with other programming strands. This situation continued until the launch of the BBC Music Programme on March 22nd 1965. This service broadcast classical music between 7.00 am and 6.30 pm daily.

While the Third Programme attracted a niche audience the other BBC services delivered listeners en-masse. Programmes like 'Much-Binding-in-the-Marsh', 'Take it from Here' and 'Ray's a Laugh' proved to be hugely popular with the British public.

'Much-Binding-in-the-Marsh' starred Kenneth Horne and Richard Murdoch as senior staff in a fictional RAF station. Over the years the station became a country club and finally a newspaper. The show had a chequered broadcasting career and was broadcast on BBC radio from 1944 to 1950. It transferred to Radio Luxembourg between 1950 and 1951. Then it returned to the BBC until it ended its run in 1954. One of the most fondly remembered parts of the show was the closing theme tune, which featured topical lyrics sung by members of the cast.

'Take It from Here' ran on the BBC between 1948 and 1960. It starred Jimmy Edwards, Dick Bentley and Joy Nichols. Nichols left the show in 1953 and was replaced by June Whitfield and Alma Cogan. The shows writers were Frank Muir and Denis Norden, who are credited with reinventing British post-war radio comedy. It was one of the first shows with a significant segment parodying film and book styles. The show is probably best known for a series of sketches featuring a uncouth dysfunctional family called 'The Glums'.

The Glum family were the antithesis of cosy middle class families portrayed in the media at the time. Pa Glum (Edwards) was a cantankerous old soak. His son Ron (Bentley) was a feckless layabout, despite the relentless efforts of his ambitious fiancée Eth (Whitfield). Mrs. Glum, the family matriarch was often heard incoherently in the distance. Alma Cogan, the singer, usually provided Ma Glum's off-stage noises.

'Ray's a Laugh' starring Ted Ray, was a more traditional show. It was essentially a domestic comedy with musical items. Ray's wife was played by Kitty Bluett and Fred Yule played his brother-in-law. The supporting cast included a fine array of comedy stalwarts such as Patricia Hayes, Kenneth Connor, Pat Coombs and Graham Stark. Another early cast member was a talented newcomer called Peter Sellers, who would go on to more anarchic humour later in his career. 'Ray's a Laugh' ran from 1949 until January 1961.

1947 was an important year for the BBC but it didn't start too well for them. A hard winter and a fuel crisis forced the Corporation to take drastic action. They suspended the Third Programme and amalgamated the Light Programme and Home Service for a short period during February and March. Full daytime programming was not reinstated until April.

On November 14th the BBC celebrated their Silver Jubilee by publishing a pamphlet called 'Twenty Five Years of British Broadcasting'. They also transmitted a number of special programmes. On November 20th the BBC broadcast the wedding of Her Royal Highness Princess Elizabeth (the future Queen Elizabeth II) to Lieutenant Philip Mountbatten (the future Prince Philip, Duke of Edinburgh), at Westminster Abbey.

The International Broadcasting Company (IBC) stations didn't return after the war. Changes in French media law meant that private stations couldn't operate with the same freedom as they had done before the war. In 1947, Leonard Plugge and Fernand Legrande held discussions regarding the possible revival of Radio Normandy's English Service. However these talks were never concluded satisfactorily and the service never returned.

Instead the IBC headquarters in Portland Place became one of the best independent recording studios in Britain. During the 1960s and 1970s the studios were used by some of the biggest recording artists in the world.

Radio Luxembourg remained in the hands of Allied forces for some time after the war. Special programmes were broadcast for the American occupying forces. It was also strongly rumoured that Winston Churchill wanted to use the transmitter facilities as a propaganda weapon against the Soviet Union. This plan never came to fruition and Radio Luxembourg was handed back to its owners during the summer of 1946.

When Luxembourg returned it was business as usual and Stephen Williams resumed his role as manager of the English service. Transmissions had restarted on the same pre-war long wave frequency. Unfortunately Radio Luxembourg found it difficult to attract English advertisers and the broadcasts were gradually reduced and replaced by other languages.

On July 2nd 1951, the English programmes were transferred to a less powerful medium wave frequency - 208 metres. These transmissions could only be received satisfactorily in Britain during the hours of darkness, when the signal was able to bounce off the ionosphere and reach the United Kingdom.

Geoffrey Everett was in charge by this time as Stephen Williams had moved to the BBC to become a producer. The station adopted the slogan '208 – Your station of the stars', which referred to the performers heard on the station.

Despite the relegation to medium wave, this became a golden period for Radio Luxembourg. Popular programmes at the time included 'Dr Kildare', 'Dan Dare – Pilot of the Future' and the 'Top Twenty Programme'. The latter was a show featuring the best selling records of the week. This was the first time such a programme had been attempted in Europe. The Top Twenty Programme became Radio Luxembourg's most popular show and received around 1,500 letters a week.

Sponsored programmes made up the majority of airtime. Quiz programmes such as 'Take Your Pick' and 'Double Your Money' proved immensely popular. The Ovaltineys also returned to enthral a new generation of children.

Halfway during the decade Luxembourg's English service became mainly a music station. Numerous presenters fronted shows sponsored by record companies such as EMI, Decca and Capitol.

The move to nightly music shows coincided with the introduction of the transistor radio and the emergence of youth culture and Rock 'n' Roll. The opportunity to hear such music on BBC radio was limited to a Sunday afternoon review of the current charts and a Saturday morning programme called 'The Saturday Skiffle Club'. The show was later renamed 'Saturday Club' when the skiffle craze ended.

However Radio Luxembourg fully embraced the new musical phenomenon. Teenagers all over Europe would listen under the bedclothes to 'The Great 208', which offered a non stop diet of popular tunes in marked contrast to the sparse offerings of the BBC. Listening to Radio Luxembourg could be a frustrating experience for the dedicated music fan. The sponsored shows aimed to publicise as many of their new releases as possible. Therefore the disc jockeys never played a complete record and would usually fade it halfway through. Another problem was the famous 'Luxembourg fade'. Luxembourg's signal suffered from atmospheric interference and would often fade in and out for seconds, or even minutes, at a time. So if the disc jockeys didn't fade your favourite record, the atmosphere would do it instead. Tuning to the station required endless patience and almost constant readjustment.

BBC radio continued to have some huge successes through the early part of the fifties. Woman's Hour is a magazine programme that began on the Light Programme in 1946 and still continues today. The programme contained reports, interviews and debates on health, education, cultural topics and short-run drama serials. Although aimed ostensibly at women, Woman's Hour also featured items of general interest. The programme switched to a morning slot in 1991 where it has remained ever since.

Alistair Cooke began his long running series 'Letter from America' on March 24th 1946. Originally born in Salford, Lancashire, Cooke emigrated to America shortly before the outbreak of the Second World War. Cooke suggested to the BBC a series of 15-minute talks for British listeners on life in America. A prototype, 'Mainly about Manhattan', was broadcast intermittently from 1938 but was dropped when war broke out. After that, Cooke broadcast a weekly 'American Commentary' on the BBC about the war. 'Letter from America' was initially commissioned for only 13 instalments but finally came to an end 58 years (2,869 episodes) later, in March 2004.

'Down Your Way' began on December 29th 1946. The programme visited towns around the United Kingdom, spoke to residents and played their choice of music. 'Down Your Way' vividly evoked the local and regional distinctiveness of Britain as it moved around the country. Stewart MacPherson initially hosted the programme until

Richard Dimbleby replaced him in 1950. Five years later, Franklin Engelmann took over presentation duties until his death in 1972. The next presenter was Brian Johnston, who lasted until 1987. However there was a brief hiatus during Johnston's tenure. In 1975, despite then being the second most popular programme on radio, it was taken off the air as 'an economy measure'. It was subsequently brought back after thousands of listeners objected.

Whilst undoubtedly popular, the programme was not without its critics. Their view was that 'Down Your Way' portrayed an increasingly old-fashioned and rose-tinted view of Britain. The critics' opinion was that the programme concentrated too much on market towns with pre-industrial roots and ignored industrial towns and urban conurbations. From 1987, until its demise in 1992, it had a different celebrity host every week. The guest presenters would visit a place of significance in their own lives - effectively turning it into 'Down My Way' and blending it into the then-emerging celebrity culture.

'Listen with Mother' was a programme featuring stories, songs and nursery rhymes for children under five (and their mothers). It was broadcast on the Light Programme for fifteen minutes every weekday afternoon at 1.45, just before Woman's Hour. The theme music, which became synonymous with the programme, was the Berceuse from Gabriel Fauré's 'Dolly Suite for piano duet, Op. 56'. The programme's opening phrase 'Are you sitting comfortably? Then I'll begin' etched itself into the British consciousness and is still recited by people who probably never heard the original programme. At its peak, 'Listen with Mother' had an audience of over a million. Like Woman's Hour, it was subsequently transferred to the Home Service. The programme lasted until 1982

The BBC decided to try out an American radio format – the 'Soap Opera'. However they called these programmes 'Serial Dramas'. 'Mrs Dale's Diary' was the first major example of this type to appear on the BBC. The storyline featured a doctor's wife, Mrs. Mary Dale and her husband Jim. Each episode began with a brief narrative spoken by Mrs. Dale as if she were writing her diary. The Dales lived at Virginia Lodge in the fictional London suburb of Parkwood Hill. 'Mrs Dale's Diary' began on the Light Programme on 5 January 1948, and subsequently transferred to the newly formed Radio 2 in 1967, where it ran until 25 April 1969. A new episode was broadcast each weekday afternoon, with a repeat the following morning.

'The Archers' was first transmitted in the Midlands area as a pilot series on May 29th 1950. The BBC decided to commission the series for a longer national run. The series began on New Years Day 1951 and continues to this day. In fact it is now the world's longest running soap opera. The programme was originally billed as "an everyday story of country folk", but is now described by the BBC as "contemporary drama in a rural setting. 'The Archers' is set in the fictional village of Ambridge in the equally fictional county of Borsetshire. Borsetshire is said to situated between the real counties of Worcestershire and Warwickshire,

Unlike some soap operas, episodes of 'The Archers' portray events taking place on the date of broadcast, allowing many topical subjects to be included. Real-life events that can be readily predicted in advance are often written into the script, such as the FIFA World Cup or the annual Oxford Farming Conference. On some occasions, scenes recorded at these events are planned and edited into episodes shortly before transmission. However some significant but unforeseen events require scenes to be rewritten and rerecorded at short notice.

The BBC transmitted several other landmark broadcasts during the 1950s. The funeral of King George VI was broadcast on BBC Radio and Television on February 15th 1951. Then there was the coronation of his daughter, Queen Elizabeth II, on June 2nd 1953. The first ball-by-ball Test Match Special appeared on BBC radio on June 30th 1957.

Undoubtedly the comedy hit of the 1950s was a programme that starred Peter Sellers, Harry Secombe, Spike Milligan and, initially, Michael Bentine. The first series, broadcast between May and September 1951, was titled 'Crazy People'. After Bentine's departure at the end of the first series, the show was renamed 'The Goon Show'.

The show's chief creator and main writer was Spike Milligan. The scripts mixed preposterous storylines with surreal humour, puns, catchphrases and peculiar sound effects. Many elements of the show satirised various aspects of life in Britain at the time. The talented cast complemented the bizarre scripts by utilising a wide range of increasingly wacky voices to portray the eccentric characters. It could be said that 'The Goon Show' was an audio cartoon. That is creating cartoons by means of sounds, voices and sound effects

The Goon Show remained popular long after the show finished in 1960 and is continuously repeated at regular intervals. A special one off edition of the show was broadcast as part of the BBC's 50th anniversary celebrations. Generations of subsequent British comedians cite the show as one of their main influences

'Hancock's Half-Hour' *was* less fanciful than the Goons but equally influential. Comedian Tony Hancock was the star of the show. The series broke with the variety tradition which was then dominant in British radio comedy. Instead of the normal mix of sketches, guest stars and musical interludes, the show's humour derived from characters and situations developed in a half-hour storyline. It could be said that Hancock's Half Hour was the first British situation comedy.

Hancock played an exaggerated and much poorer version of his own character that lived at the dilapidated 23 Railway Cuttings in East Cheam. His sidekicks or, more often than not, his own embarrassing shortcomings constantly thwart Hancock's fanciful ambitions in life. Sid James played Hancock's criminally-inclined friend and Bill Kerr appeared as Hancock's dim-witted Australian lodger. From the third series, Hattie Jaques played Griselda Pugh, who was Hancock's secretary and Sid's occasional girlfriend. The show started on radio in 1954 and transferred to television two years later Hancock was the first British comedian to make the transition from radio to television.

Radio stations in the U.S.A. began experiments with broadcasting on VHF (very high frequency) using FM (frequency modulation) in January 1941. The first BBC VHF-FM radio transmissions started on May 2nd 1955 from Wrotham in Kent. These transmissions offered better quality and were less susceptible to the types of interference often encountered on medium and long wave broadcasts. Medium wave transmissions frequently suffered interference from Continental stations after dark. Long Wave broadcasts experienced interference from unsuppressed electrical motors, thermostats etc.

This new service brought high fidelity radio to around 13 million potential listeners in London and the South East of England. The BBC gradually introduced more high power transmitters followed by many low power relay stations that filled in some significant pockets of poor reception. All the VHF-FM transmissions were initially in mono

The first stereo test transmissions began on 28th August 1962. The BBC used the Third Programme transmitter at Wrotham, which remained the only source of stereo radio for some years. The problem for the BBC was the distribution of stereo to its transmitters. At that time the organisation relied totally on the GPO's network of landlines for programme distribution and stereo required not one but two such lines. Also, these lines had to be carefully matched in terms of their quality and their length, and this proved to be difficult.

The BBC eventually solved the problem by using a system they called Pulse Code Modulation. This system could convert 13 audio channels into one digital bit stream. This stream could be carried easily using the sort of link that carried television pictures. The BBC added stereo capability to Radios 2 & 4 in 1973 and stereo radio finally began to extend across the British Isles.

The BBC reorganised their three networks on September 30th 1957. The majority of the Home Service's lighter content transferred to the Light Programme. The Third Programme was renamed the BBC Third Network and cultural programmes were reduced from 40 to 24 hours a week. The extra hours were used to incorporate the Home Service's adult education content and the Home and Light's sports coverage.

Despite its prominent position for nearly four decades, radio's popularity declined swiftly during the 1950s. The main reason for this was undoubtedly the ascendancy of radio's electronic progeny - television.

During the early part of the 1950s the BBC concentrated most of its efforts on radio. In 1950 there were 12 million radio-only licences and only 350,000 combined radio and TV licences. The BBC budget for television was a fraction of the radio one. However the Coronation of Queen Elizabeth II on June 2nd 1953 was a turning point. This was the first time that a television audience exceeded the size of a radio audience. An estimated 20 million TV viewers saw the young Queen crowned. The following year saw the amount of combined sound and vision licences rise to over three million. The television age had arrived in Britain.

9

Radio Down Under

In this chapter we look at the development of radio in the Southern hemisphere. At the beginning of the 20th century, Australia was a newly federated country. The new Government realised that the broadcasting spectrum should be regulated and wireless telegraphy quickly came under their control. The Wireless Telegraphy Act of 1905 was introduced and since then broadcasting in Australia has remained the responsibility of federal governments. In this same year Marconi's company built Australia's first two-way wireless telegraphy station at Queenscliff in Victoria. Marconi and its main competitor Telefunken amalgamated to form Amalgamated Wireless (Australasia) Ltd. in 1913.

That same year, The AWA established the Marconi Telefunken College of Telegraphy (later re-named the Marconi School of Wireless). This establishment made a valuable contribution during the two world wars. During times of conflict there is always a tremendous need for radio communications and Australia was able to maintain a high level of expertise. This has been attributed mainly to the effectiveness of the Marconi School of Wireless.

After the 'Titanic' tragedy in 1912, many nations around the world agreed to provide coastal communication services to ensure the safety of seafarers. The first Australian coastal radio station was established in Melbourne in 1912. More stations followed and by 1914 there were 19 coastal stations around the Australian mainland. At first the stations communicated with Morse telegraphy. Short wave transmission and two-way radio telephone were introduced after the Second World War. In the 1990s, satellite technologies were introduced and this resulted in a steep decline in radio traffic.

After the First World War there were 900 radio amateurs in Australia. The first 'broadcast' in Australia was organised by George Fisk of Amalgamated Wireless on August 19th 1919. Fisk arranged for the National Anthem to be broadcast from one building to another at the end of a lecture he'd given on the new medium to the Royal Society of New South Wales.

The radio manufacturing industry in Australia lobbied the Government for the introduction of radio broadcasting in these early years. In May 1923, the Government finally called a conference which led to the sealed set regulations. On payment of a fee, people received a radio that was set to the frequency of the stations they had subscribed to. 2FC in Sydney was the first to be licensed on July 1st 1923 but its opponent 2SB was first to go to air.

2SB began on November 13th 1923. The first programme was a concert featuring a soprano, a bass, a contralto, a cellist, a baritone and quartet. The baritone, George Saunders, was the station's first announcer. 2FC followed with its first public broadcast on December 5th 1923. After several months of transmission it was evident that listeners were confused by the similarly sounding call signs of 2SB and 2FC. So in March 1924, 2SB changed its name and became 2BL.

The sealed set scheme wasn't popular; only 1400 people took out sealed set licences in the first 6 months of 1924. It was quite easy to avoid the licence fee by building your own set or modifying one you'd bought to receive more than one station. The radio industry proposed an alternative two-tiered system – A and B licences. The Australian Government accepted this compromise proposal in July 1924. The 'A' licences were largely financed by listeners' licence fees, imposed and collected by the Government. 'B' class stations would have to generate their own revenue through advertising. 'This system was an amalgam of the British and American structures and Australia ended up with the parallel system of a national network alongside a commercial network.

By the end of 1924 the number of listener licences was close to 40,000 and had doubled to 80,000 by the end of 1925. The first 'B' class station on air was 2BE in November 1924. However it closed down in 1929 so the oldest surviving commercial station is 2UE, which went on air on Australia Day 1925. South Australia's first stations were 5CL (an 'A' class station), which started on November 20th 1924, and 5DN (a commercial station), which went live on February 24th 1925.

The British Government nationalized radio in 1926 by buying out the British Broadcasting Company and forming the British Broadcasting Corporation. That same year, the Australian Government held a Royal Commission into Wireless. The Government did not immediately follow the British lead but they did encourage the 'A' class stations to amalgamate in order to maximise efficiencies and maintain standards.

In 1929, the Australian Government nationalised the transmission facilities. After calling for tenders, the Government granted a three-year contract to the Australian Broadcasting Company, consisting of Fullers Theatres, Greater Union Theatres and music publishers J. Albert & Son. They were to take over all A-class stations and produce programmes on a national basis. Initially the ABC was to be allowed to broadcast advertisements but this was dropped from the final Bill. Instead, it was funded by radio listeners' licences. Licence fees for radio and TV were finally dropped in the seventies and ABC's funding now comes from Federal Government appropriation. When their contract ran out in 1932, the Australian Broadcasting Company was nationalised and the Australian Broadcasting Commission was established. This meant that Australia had 12 stations run by the ABC and 43 commercial stations.

Australia was a leader in the use of short wave broadcasting to transmit overseas. In 1927, Amalgamated Wireless (Australasia) conducted a series of transmissions to Britain. These regular broadcasts were heralded by a kookaburra's laugh - a practice that's still used by Radio Australia today. Radio Australia was formally incorporated as part of the ABC in 1939.

The Federation of Australian Radio Broadcasters was established in 1930. This was an industry body with a remit to look after and promote commercial radio interests. In 1934, the commercial radio sector pulled off a great scoop when it won the rights to broadcast commentary of cricket matches between England and Australia. The Test Match series was being played in the United Kingdom that year and this greatly boosted the amount of radios and licences purchased

In New Zealand, radio licensing was first introduced in 1923. Stations sprang up in all parts of the country. These included 1YA and 1YB in Auckland, 2YB and 2YK in Wellington and 3AC in Christchurch. Radio manufacturers and shops selling musical instruments and sheet music ran many of these stations. These outfits were often called 'trade' stations. Overseas radio manufacturers often supported these local businesses.

Amateur operators and radio societies also broadcast entertainment programmes regularly. The Radio Broadcasting Company of New Zealand was established as a national operation in 1925. This was after an earlier plan by the NZ Co-Operative Dairy Company to operate a station aimed at dairy farmers was rejected.

Call signs were allocated by the government and divided New Zealand into four radio districts: 1 was allocated to Auckland (roughly a line between King Country, Taupo, Whakatane and all points north). Wellington and the rest of the North Island plus Nelson, Marlborough and the Chatham Islands were allotted call signs beginning with 2. The call sign 3 was assigned to Christchurch (Canterbury as far south as South Canterbury, plus Buller and Westland). The suffix 4 was allocated to Dunedin and the rest of the South Island.

1931 would prove to be a pivotal year in the early history of radio broadcasting in New Zealand. That year, royalty disagreements shut down numerous stations and the Napier earthquake knocked several more stations off air. However the most important change was the expiration of the Radio Broadcasting Company's agreement. It was not renewed and the government established the New Zealand Broadcasting Board instead.

The NZBC pressed ahead with its own extension of radio coverage. High-powered transmitters were ordered for use in Auckland, Wellington, Christchurch, and Dunedin and were sited at various points to achieve best coverage. New Zealand's main broadcasting problem was reaching the relatively small pockets of population concentrated in the fertile areas that lay among mountain ranges. The Board decided to give financial aid to a number of private broadcasting stations operating in areas where reception of the Board's stations was unsatisfactory.

However the New Zealand Broadcasting Board's tenure was brief. In 1935 the country had gone to the polls and resolutely returned its first Labour Government. One of the first legislative measures passed was the Broadcasting Act 1936, which came into force on July 1st. One of the main provisions of the legislation was the abolition of the New Zealand Broadcasting Board. All the rights, property, liabilities, and engagements of the Board were transferred to the Crown. As a result, for the foreseeable future, broadcasting was to be administered as a Government Department.

Undoubtedly the most controversial aspect of the Broadcasting Act was the prohibition of advertising, except by commercial stations controlled by the government. Deprived of their revenue stream, all privately owned commercial stations were forced to close down.

Despite the government's virtual broadcasting monopoly, listeners in New Zealand could hear a wide variety of stations from other sources. At night stations from Australia, Hawaii, California and even Asia could be easily heard as there were hardly any local stations to listen to. Stations such as 2FC in Sydney, KFI in Los Angeles and KGU in Honolulu proved to be very popular.

In Australia the expansion of radio continued rapidly. By the early 1940s there were about 130 commercial stations and a similar number of ABC stations available. The ABC had national commitments including news, education, parliamentary broadcasting and culture. The commercial stations were much more local and community-orientated in nature.

At the outbreak of World War Two, radio was viewed as the main information source of war news. For the first time, Australians could hear, rather than just read, reports from the battle fronts. Australian radio networks sent correspondents to all areas of combat and reports were recorded and sent back to Australia. Australian radio programmes were also sent to the troops. Music, drama and entertainment were also very important throughout the war years as a way of keeping up morale.

On February 2nd 1942, Australia's first nationally sponsored morning serial was broadcast across a network of stations. 'Big Sister' originated from 2UW in Sydney, although the scripts were American. The show, sponsored by Lever and Kitchen, was heard five mornings a week. Throughout its five-year run it was the top rated daytime show and was the forerunner of many other daytime serials in that genre.

The years after the Second World War are considered to be radio's golden era. Radio drama became very popular in Australia. The most popular radio dramas were 'Blue Hills', 'The Lawsons' and 'Dad and Dave'. Australian children had their own radio programme called the 'Argonauts Club'. The Argonauts Club ran for 30 years from 1941 to 1971. Over 50 000 Australian children became members of the club during that era.

Many American formats were adapted for Australian radio. The Lux Radio Theatre began in Australia on March 19th 1939, after five successful years on American radio. The series of one-hour plays were transmitted at 8pm on Sunday nights, which was peak listening time. Other American shows adapted for Australia included 'Inner Sanctum Mysteries', 'The Falcon', 'Dragnet', 'The Witches Tale', 'Nightbeat' and 'The Shadow'.

The Broadcasting & Television Act had originally been enacted in 1942 but a major amendment was introduced in 1948. This was to introduce a regulatory body - the Australian Broadcasting Control Board. The new authority maintained there was no room for new stations on the AM band so experimental FM broadcasts began.

There was another major amendment in 1956 to introduce television and a further inquiry into FM in 1957. However the commercial operators were unwilling to invest in the new infrastructure that would be required. Planned FM services were shelved and eventually the Australian Broadcasting Control Board authorised the use of the international VHF FM band for television in 1961.

The closure of the FM experimental stations, together with the Australian Broadcasting Control Board's recalcitrant position on AM broadcasts, meant that no new competition came onto the scene. There was widespread dissatisfaction with the Government for not introducing FM quality broadcasting. This emanated mainly from people who wanted to hear 'fine music' (classical or jazz) on the airwaves.

In 1961, Dr. Neil Runcie formed the Listener's Society of New South Wales. Their major intention was to establish subscriber-supported FM music stations. This concept had had some success in the USA with the Pacifica stations and a few educational FM stations.

In the same year the University of New South Wales was given a licence under the Wireless and Telegraphy Act to broadcast lectures over a non-broadcast frequency. This station was assigned the call letters VL-2UV.

These two organisations were the progenitors of a movement to provide more diversity in Australia's radio broadcasting. Ultimately this movement led to the establishment of the third tier of broadcasting in Australia, the public or community sector.

The third prong of this movement came from Australia's ethnic communities. Australia had undertaken the biggest programme of immigration in the world after the Second World War. The country's population had almost doubled in 20 years. By the late sixties this large group of immigrants, many of them from non-English speaking backgrounds, was reaching political maturity. Ethnic communities were demanding a more open media.

In 1964, the Australian Broadcasting Control Board had allowed for up to 10% of broadcasting time to be in non-English languages. The commercial sector utilized this provision for revenue and stations such as 2CH and 3XY sublet airtime to ethnic groups. However as commercial radio became more competitive and format-driven, the amount of ethnic broadcasting decreased until in 1972 there were only 36 hours in six languages of ethnic broadcasting in the country.

The fourth group seeking access to the airwaves were young political activists. There was a climate of political unrest in the late sixties with people protesting against Australia's involvement in the Vietnam War. In 1971, Melbourne University students set up a pirate radio station in the Union building and broadcast anti-government messages. It was only on air for a few hours before Federal Police broke in and confiscated the transmitting equipment. That same year, the weak response to the Springbok rugby tour demonstrations led Brisbane students to look at forming their own radio station. This eventually became 4ZZZ.

In the early part of 1972, the Australian Broadcasting Control Board held another broadcasting inquiry. One of the recommendations of this report was the introduction of public access broadcasting. This differed from the other two radio sectors because of community involvement in both the management and programming of the station. The 'community' could be a geographically defined district or a society of special interest. These stations were to be non-profit and community owned. They wouldn't receive government funding and were only allowed limited advertising.

The other main initiative from the 1972 inquiry by the ABCB was the introduction of FM broadcasting. However this was planned for the UHF band rather than the internationally used VHF band. This was suggested by the radio manufacturing industry who wanted to sell sets that were only usable in Australia.

By the time the recommendations were implemented in the mid-seventies, common sense had prevailed. The UHF proposals had been rejected in favour of the more popular VHF band. The first use of FM in Australia was for non-profit community-based public broadcasting. The first station on FM was 2MBS in Sydney, which started in the latter part of 1974. 3MBS in Melbourne followed the following summer. Both stations had a 'fine music' format. The ABC entered the medium in 1976 with the establishment of ABC-FM based in Adelaide.

VL-5UV in Adelaide is often cited as Australia's first public access station. The station, which made its first broadcast in June 1972, was established as a direct educational outreach of the University of Adelaide. At this stage its wavelength was off the AM band due to legal requirements and was restricted to twelve broadcast hours per week. VL-5UV could not really be described as a public/community broadcaster at this point. It did not have community access or ethnic programmes. Its programming was strictly didactic; lectures were recorded and rebroadcast later.

VL-5UV was broadcast from studios based in the Barr Smith Library complex. The station's initial funding was made possible by a bequest to the University of $100,000. This was from the estate of Kenneth Stirling, who was a graduate of the University. Stirling had stipulated the money was to be used for an educational initiative. The quality of training and experience available to volunteers at the station was quickly recognised as 5UV 'graduates' were employed by the ABC and the commercial networks.

VL-5UV wanted to expand the station's programming and move to the access and participation model that was to eventually characterise public broadcasting. However they were not licensed to do so and had to wait for legislation that would permit them to do this.

The Wireless & Telegraph Act was eventually introduced in 1974. The new legislation meant that that VL-5UV could finally move into the AM band. They switched to 530 kHz, which was later upgraded to 531 KHz. The station's name was shortened to 5UV at this point and many specialist and ethnic groups were given airtime.

5UV gained an FM outlet in October 2001 and AM broadcasting ceased the following January. Gradually the station became more independent of the university and is now located in its own premises. The station adopted a 2-part name change process. Radio 5UV is now known as Radio Adelaide, following a provisional period known as 5UV Radio Adelaide.

The commercial sector had been unwilling to commit to FM broadcasts when the spectrum was first offered in the early 1970s. Therefore they were overlooked when FM was inaugurated and the spectrum went to public and community broadcasters instead. The commercial operators swiftly realised the error of their ways and began to petition the Australian government. They wanted their AM stations to have the right to simulcast on FM but this was not accepted.

Instead, in 1980, the Government offered a limited number of FM licences. Two in Melbourne and Sydney and one each in each other capital city, the same as in 1924 when the 'A' class licences were first introduced. However these licences went to new companies rather than the existing stations. The new FM commercial stations swiftly became profitable and became the ratings leader in most markets.

After much lobbying, the Government allowed a chosen few AM stations to convert to FM. A common trait of the eighties was financial rationalism - a concern for putting an economic value on everything. In broadcasting this meant that the broadcast spectrum was seen as an asset that had monetary value. This led to an auction of the FM frequencies and the resultant bidding war to win the right to convert severely affected the economies of the commercial sector. In addition, the radio industry got ensnared in the media buying frenzy that accompanied the widespread entrepreneurial boom during the latter part of the eighties. As a result, many stations got into financial difficulties and changed hands.

A good example of a station changing hands was 3EON in Melbourne. They were the first commercial FM radio station in Australia, beating Fox FM to the title by two weeks. Eon FM's inaugural FM broadcast took place on July 11th 1980. At first the station had no playlist and deliberately avoided Top 40 songs. They widely publicised that Eon FM would feature songs that "would not be played elsewhere".

Although the station out-performed other FM stations it was comprehensibly beaten by the AM stations. The management was worried about this and shareholders were asked to invest another $1 million between them only a year after the station was launched. Shortly afterwards, Eon FM abandoned the album rock format and began playing Top 40 records instead. This changed the station's fortunes and it eventually topped the ratings in 1985. The following year, 3EON FM was sold to the Triple M network and eventually rebranded to 3MMM on November 27th 1988.

As the 1980s became the 1990s, many stations were purchased by large networks. In turn the networks would be swallowed up by other predatory networks. 1992 saw a monopolistic arrangement take place whereby the Austereo network purchased the Triple M network owned by the Hoyts Group. Then Austereo was purchased by the Village Roadshow media company. This deal was unpopular due to the fierce rivalry between the two radio networks. Village Roadshow and Hoyts were also direct competitors in the film industry.

In March 2011, Southern Cross Media launched a takeover bid of the Austereo Group. The following month, shareholders of the Austereo Group accepted the takeover bid, giving Southern Cross Media a 90% share in the company. Southern Cross Media and Austereo officially merged in July 2011 to form Southern Cross Austereo

The new group now has two distinct radio networks amongst its media portfolio. The Today Network - a popular music format targeted at 18-39 year olds, using various Today Network brands in metropolitan areas along with the Star FM, Hot FM and Sea FM brands in regional areas. The other network is Triple M – a talk and adult contemporary music format aimed at over 35s, mainly on the AM and heritage FM stations, as well as Triple M, Gold FM, Mix FM and Radio West in Western Australia.

Australia has had an extensive commercial radio network since the 1920s. However, as we've heard previously, radio in New Zealand remained firmly under the aegis of the government. The National Broadcasting Service, and its successor - the New Zealand Broadcasting Corporation, had been operating since 1936. No privately owned station had been allowed to operate for over thirty years. In the mid 1960s, the impetus for privately owned commercial radio came from a rather surprising area.

The genesis of modern day commercial radio in New Zealand took the form of a group of radio pirates in international waters off the coast of Auckland. Radio Hauraki transmitted from studios aboard the ships 'Tiri' and its successor 'Tiri II'. The station officially started broadcasting on December 4th 1966 and its Americanised top 40 music format was immensely successful. Radio Hauraki's success forced the Government to create the New Zealand Broadcasting Authority in 1968. This Authority issued the first two private commercial broadcasting licences on March 24th 1970. One of the successful applicants was Radio Hauraki.

Unfortunately for the proponents of commercial radio, the allocation of licences was slower than expected. By 1972 only five private stations were on the air in New Zealand. In response to public pressure, the 1974 Labour government pushed through legislation that split the state-run New Zealand Broadcasting Corporation into three distinct sectors. One of these was Radio New Zealand – an amalgamation of commercial and non-commercial stations and networks. At this point more commercial stations were introduced into markets around New Zealand.

In 1981, new legislation allowed the newly formed Broadcasting Tribunal to issue FM broadcasting warrants for the first time. This led to 22 private and 37 government owned commercial radio stations in 1984. However it was the introduction of the Radio Broadcasting Act in 1989 that generated the biggest expansion. All available frequencies around the country went up for tender and new ownership groups were formed. Commercial radio in New Zealand became arguably the most deregulated in the world. By April 1993, over 200 new frequencies were active and the increase continued exponentially. In 2004, over 700 frequencies were available for broadcast on AM and FM in New Zealand. This was possibly the largest number per capita anywhere in the world.

The reforms in radio structure were not restricted to the commercial sector as the government reviewed its own assets. 'Ruthanasia', a combination of 'Ruth' and 'euthanasia', was the deprecatory appellation given to the period of free-market economic reform conducted by the New Zealand Government during the latter half of the 1990s. The 'Ruth' in Ruthanasia referred to the then Minister of Finance, Ruth Richardson. As a result of this reform, the government's commercial radio operations were sold to a conglomerate for $89 million in 1996. The Radio Network (TRN) was a partnership between Independent News and Media and Clear Channel.

Other private ownership groups were quick to react to the formation of this media giant. In early 1997, Energy Enterprises merged with Radio Pacific and Canadian-based CanWest purchased the Frader Group. In May 1999, the Radio Pacific-Energy Enterprises group completed a takeover of Radio Otago and evolved into RadioWorks Ltd. Finally in May 2000, CanWest announced the successful purchase of RadioWorks and the commercial radio battle was down to just two major competitors: The Radio Network and CanWest Global. Both groups continued their acquisition spree and by 2005, TRN and CanWest owned or controlled over 350 frequencies in New Zealand.

These mergers and acquisitions would become a regular occurrence elsewhere in the world and, despite the consolidation; the radio industry within the Australasia region remains vibrant and healthy.

10

Radio Fights Back

In Britain, television really began to catch on when the first commercial station began on September 22nd 1955. The new Independent Television Authority (ITA) began its broadcasts with live coverage of an opening ceremony and banquet at the Guildhall in London. After the Guildhall banquet, the main programmes got under way. They included half an hour of drama excerpts, news bulletins, a variety show and a boxing match. Epilogue, a five-minute religious programme, ended the evening's transmissions at 2300 BST.

The first commercial came a little more than an hour into the schedule. Viewers saw a tube of Gibbs SR toothpaste in a block of ice, with a voice over pronouncing it 'a tingling fresh toothpaste for teeth and gums'. There were another 23 advertisements during the evening, promoting products ranging from Cadbury's chocolate to Esso petrol.

However BBC Radio staged an effective spoiling tactic that managed to upstage the launch of ITV. The BBC broadcast a controversial episode of 'The Archers' featuring the death of Grace Archer, a leading character in the serial. The episode pulled in an audience of 20 million and generated a lot of column inches in the newspapers. The BBC has always maintained that this was coincidental and not a deliberate plan to divert attention from the opening night of commercial television.

The arrival of commercial television created great controversy. Some compared its arrival to that of the great plague. Winston Churchill was unimpressed and described it as 'a tupenny Punch and Judy show'. The BBC, hindered by its dependency on a licence fee fixed by the Government, saw its audience share drop to 28%. Nevertheless, competition gave the BBC a necessary jolt, forcing it to revamp its drama and news presentations.

In America, radio also played second fiddle to television. By 1950, more than 4 million television sets had been sold and the radio set had lost its valued place in American living rooms to the new arrival.

Radio stations found it difficult to retain staff as sales people and programme personnel defected en masse to the new medium.

Perhaps the biggest threat posed to American radio by television was financial. Advertisers were seduced by the newer, sexier medium and gradually reduced their radio budget. However, unlike its signals, radio did not fade away. Station owners simply adjusted their tactics to cope with the new economic realities. With network programmes on the decline, most local stations couldn't afford to finance large variety shows or dramas so they turned to a cheaper alternative instead. They broadcast pre-recorded music linked by live personalities, or disc jockeys, as they later became known.

Many station owners realised that the days of broadcasting to a substantial amount of listeners were over and elected to aim their transmissions at a niche audience instead. By 'narrowcasting', they identified target audiences and created formats to specifically appeal to those listeners. By the end of the decade, various musical formats such as rock 'n' roll, jazz, classical and country had proliferated.

A strong local identity was essential and many stations seized every opportunity to get involved in local affairs. They increased local news bulletins and frequently publicised events in their area. This localness, combined with specialist programming, helped to save American radio from its television-induced decline.

The new style of American radio featuring music laced together by a fast talking Disc Jockey proved to be extremely popular. The success of this new broadcast format was boosted by the emergence of rock 'n' roll. As older listeners transferred their allegiance to television, youngsters replaced them as the core radio audience.

Listeners in Europe had to wait a while before they were able to experience the non-stop diet of pop music that proliferated in America. The BBC only had a limited amount of suitable programmes each week and Luxembourg's schedule was full of sponsored record company shows.

In 1958, a group of pioneers circumvented European broadcasting regulations by transmitting from ships or fixed maritime structures in international waters. These offshore stations, or 'pirates' as they became known, were able to exploit a loophole in maritime law.

A country's jurisdiction only extended as far as territorial waters. In most cases this was three miles out from the coast. In international waters a vessel need only recognise the laws of the country whose flag it sailed under. If the law of the flag state had no objection to international marine broadcasting then the ship could broadcast quite freely and legally.

The idea was not new by any means, as this had been done twenty-five years earlier in May 1933. The first 'pirate' offshore radio station was broadcast from the steam ship 'City of Panama', a floating gambling casino off the shores of California.

RKXR was permitted to transmit non-commercial programmes on 815 KHz with a power of 500 watts. However, when the ship started broadcasting it had an output power of 5,000 watts and pumped out popular music and commercials. The salt-water pathway ensured a very strong signal in Los Angeles but caused severe interference to legally licensed land-based stations. RKXR was a hit with listeners and advertisers but the positive reaction to the station caused a flurry of diplomatic activity and action was taken to close it. By August the ship was towed into Los Angeles harbour and no more was heard of the station.

A few stations broadcast from man-made structures such as old army and navy forts in the Thames estuary. Radio and TV Noordzee, a Dutch pirate, even went as far as building their own platform known as REM Island.

Europe's first 'offshore' station was a Danish pirate called Radio Mercur, which started regular transmissions on August 2nd 1958. However the station was soon joined by other ships and during it's heyday in the mid 1960s there were at least a dozen similar operations pumping out music from international waters in the North Sea.

Stations like Radio Veronica in the Netherlands and Radio London in Britain proved immensely popular with the listeners. They were only silenced when the various European Governments introduced legislation to outlaw them. These laws made it illegal for any citizen to work for, supply goods to or, more importantly, advertise on any such station.

The British version, 'The Marine Offences Act', was introduced on Monday, August 14th 1967. Most stations could not survive without advertising revenue and reluctantly complied with the law. However some stations such as Radio Caroline, the first British pirate, remained defiant. Radio Caroline continued to broadcast for some years after the Marine Broadcasting Offences Act became law in the United Kingdom.

Despite the introduction of these laws there were two fairly lengthy periods when more than one organisation was willing to deliberately flout them and broadcast from sea. As mentioned previously, Radio Caroline continued to broadcast sporadically until 1990.

The most infamous offshore station of the 1970s was Radio Northsea International, which broadcast from the coast of Holland until the Dutch government introduced their anti-pirate legislation in 1974. This station regularly made the news when events on board led to fire bomb attacks and attempted hijackings.

There was another golden offshore period in the mid '80s when Laser 558 joined Caroline in International waters. This station was launched in May 1984 by a consortium of British and American business and broadcasting executives, some of whom have never been named. Laser 558 used disc jockeys recruited from the USA. Within months the station had gained a sizeable audience, popular because of its non stop music format. However poor management and lack of advertising starved the station off the air in late 1985. In 1986 an attempt was made to return as Laser Hot Hits, but the same problems arose.

The British Government realised that outlawing the offshore stations would be hugely unpopular and unlikely to win them any votes at the next election. Therefore they persuaded the BBC to introduce a replacement. On June 30th 1967, Edward Short, the then Postmaster General, announced in Parliament that the BBC would open their new 'pop channel' in the autumn. A month later, BBC Director of Radio, Frank Gillard, announced plans to 'kill off' the Light Programme, Home Service and Third Programme. In future it would be 'Radio by Numbers'.

Radio One, the new pop music network, was launched on the morning of Saturday, September 30th 1967. The other networks also received a revamp. The Light Programme became Radio Two and the classical Third Programme was renamed Radio Three. The oldest channel, the speech-based Home service, became Radio Four.

At Broadcasting House, Paul Hollingdale opened the BBC Light Programme for the final time at 5.30AM on 30th September with 'Breakfast Special'. The studios were packed with staff and members of the press. The first Radio One Controller Robin Scott moved to studio 'A' to prepare for the takeover from Paul Hollingdale. Just a few seconds before 7am, Scott announced, "Ten seconds to go.... stand by for switching...five, four, three, Radio 2, Radio 1, GO!"

The first DJ was Tony Blackburn, who presented the new show 'Daily Disc Delivery'. The first record played was 'Flowers in the Rain' by The Move. The Bee Gees became the first live group to appear on the new network when they were guests on 'Saturday Club', at 10am.

However there were problems, Radio One was the only national BBC network that didn't get an FM outlet. The official reason for this exclusion was that there was not enough space on the FM dial, although there were no licensed Independent commercial stations at the time. Radio One's transmissions used the 16 existing medium wave relay transmitters of the Light Programme on 247 metres. However many parts of the country could not get a good signal. Scotland, Devon, Cornwall and several parts of Wales encountered reception problems after dark.

Many youngsters, the stations target audience, were dissatisfied about the replacement for the offshore radio stations. This was despite the fact that the majority of Radio One presenters had been recruited from the pirates. Of the 29 presenters listed on the opening schedules, only 12 had a BBC background. The amount of DJs hired at the launch far exceeded the positions available. They were all on short-term contracts and it became clear that a cull was inevitable. Eventually the numbers were whittled down and only the 'best' presenters survived.

The other problem was quite a large one for a network that was publicised as a 'non-stop pop channel'. The BBC had to observe 'needle time' regulations imposed by the Phonographic Performance Society. The corporation were only allowed to play 'commercial gramophone records' for 7 hours per day over both Radio One and Two. Therefore a lot of programmes had to be shared between the networks. In fact, on the first day only 5½ hours of programmes were broadcast on Radio 1 alone. Despite this restriction, the new station had doubled the Light Programme's audience within the first month of launch.

Radio One received the lion share of publicity leaving the Light Programme's replacement to its own devices. Radio 2 carried much of its predecessor's output but some of the old Light programme favourites were lost. Long running shows such as 'Music While You Work', the daily afternoon jazz and swing show 'Swingalong' and Sunday morning's 90-minute pop show 'Easy Beat' were all casualties of the shake up.

Although the BBC introduced these changes because they were forced to, it would be wrong to suggest that they didn't continue to refresh their radio output throughout the 1960s. Sir Hugh Greene became Director General in January 1960 and held the post throughout the decade. Greene believed that the corporation should reflect the social changes and attitudes of the Sixties. Greene's appointment coincided with the emergence of a new generation of British writers, journalists and performers who frequently targeted the establishment order.

The 'angry young men' were a group of playwrights and novelists who 'were disillusioned by traditional British society. A new breed of entertainer was also emerging but not from the traditional music hall / variety route. These performers were from Oxford and Cambridge University Revues and used satire as their weapon of choice. Like the 'Angry Young Men' the satirists target was the establishment. The BBC wholeheartedly encouraged these new movements and was frequently the first to employ the protagonists.

Anarchic radio comedy flourished with new programmes like 'Round the Horne' and 'I'm Sorry I'll Read That Again'. Round the Horne developed from its more traditional predecessor 'Beyond Our Ken'. Both series featured the same cast – Hugh Paddick, Betty Marsden, Bill Pertwee, Kenneth Williams and the show's front man, BBC stalwart Kenneth Horne. However 'Round the Horne' featured outlandish characters and outrageous scripts full of double entendres.

Barry Took and Marty Feldman wrote the scripts and the cast were given free reign to develop the characters. These included Charles and Fiona, a lovestruck couple engaging in stilted, polite dialogues, in scenes that parodied the romantic films of the 1940s. Then there was J. Peasemold Gruntfuttock, a disgusting and degenerate old man and Rambling Syd Rumpo, an aged folk singer. Both were played to perfection by Kenneth Williams. Probably the most fondly remembered characters were Julian and Sandy, two flamboyantly camp out-of-work actors, with Horne as their unknowing comic foil. The BBC transmitted four series of weekly episodes from 1965 until 1968. A fifth series had been commissioned, but was abandoned after Horne's untimely death in February 1969.

'I'm Sorry I'll Read That Again' *was an* irreverent comedy show, which began in 1967 and ran regularly for seven years. I'm Sorry I'll Read That Again relied heavily on the use of puns and included some jokes and catchphrases that would seem politically incorrect by the mid 1990s.

The programme is probably best known as the forerunner of two television comedy successes. The cast included John Cleese, Graeme Garden, Bill Oddie and Tim Brooke-Taylor who had all emerged from student revues. The roots of Monty Python are clearly evident, with Cleese, Chapman and Eric Idle all regular script contributors. The show's creator Humphrey Barclay would also go on to create the TV show 'Do Not Adjust Your Set', featuring the rest of the Python team. Graeme Garden, Tim Brooke Taylor and Bill Oddie would go on to create another successful television comedy – 'The Goodies'.

A strong news and current affairs strand was introduced on the Home Service. The network's flagship news programme 'Today' began on October 28th 1957. It began as a programme of 'topical talks' to give listeners a morning alternative to light music. 'Today' was initially broadcast as two 20-minute editions slotted in around the existing news bulletins.

In 1963, the programme fell under the auspices of the BBC's Current Affairs department and became more news-orientated. The two editions also became longer, and by the end of the 1960s it had become a single two-hour long programme that enveloped the news bulletins.

Jack de Manio became its main presenter in 1958. He was held in great affection by listeners but became infamous for on-air blunders and his inability to tell the time correctly. In 1970 the programme format was changed so that there were two presenters each day. In the late seventies the legendary team of John Timpson and Brian Redhead became established. Since then Libby Purves, John Humphrys, Peter Hobday, James Naughtie, Sue MacGregor, Edward Stourton, Sarah Montague, Evan Davis and Justin Webb have all fronted this broadcasting institution.

A supplemental nightly news and current affairs programme was added in 1960 and a similar lunchtime show began in 1965. Shows like 'Today', 'The World at One' and 'The World Tonight' remain a fixture today.

The BBC were also keen to get back to their roots and, in a move that hearkened back to the early days of 1923, they proposed a network of low power local stations. In December 1966 the Government granted the BBC permission to carry out a two-year experiment in local radio. These stations were to be F.M. only and would not be funded by the licence fee. Initially these stations were financed by local authorities and run by a broadcasting council staffed by local people

The first three stations in Leicester, Sheffield and Liverpool opened in November 1967, followed by five others in Nottingham, Leeds, Brighton, Durham and Stoke-on-Trent. The experiment ended in August 1969 and was deemed to be a success. However the Government were dubious that local authority financial support would be enough to maintain a permanent service and decided that the service would be rolled out using funds from an increased licence fee. Soon another twelve stations were added and today there are over forty in the BBC's local radio network.

Despite these changes the BBC's radio audience continued to fall throughout the 1970s. Undoubtedly, Television was the main cause of this as the population eagerly adopted it as their main source of information and entertainment.

Other areas of the media were also finding things tough. Newspapers found it hard to compete with the immediacy of their electronic rival. Cinemas and theatres also saw a sharp decline in attendances during this period.

The BBC had restructured its radio networks to compete with television and these changes had been largely met with approval. However the BBC's radio audience was about to fragment. Until the early 1970s, the BBC had enjoyed a legal monopoly on radio broadcasting in the UK. Up to this point it had been the policy of both major political parties that radio was to remain under the control of the BBC. Their only rivals had been sporadic broadcasts from European and offshore stations. Now there was a serious competitor on the horizon.

A change of government occurred in 1970, which saw the passing of Harold Wilson's Labour administration to Edward Heath's Conservative government. This new administration looked upon the introduction of commercial radio much more favourably. The new Minister of Post and Telecommunications, Christopher Chataway, announced a Bill to allow for the introduction of commercial radio in the United Kingdom. This service would be planned and regulated in a similar manner to the existing ITV service and would compete directly with the recently developed BBC Local Radio services.

The Sound Broadcasting Act was passed on 12 July 1972 and the Independent Television Authority (ITA) was renamed the Independent Broadcasting Authority (IBA) on that day. The authority immediately began to plan the new service and placed advertisements encouraging interested groups to apply for medium-term contracts to provide programmes in given areas.

The first major areas to be advertised were London and Glasgow. There were two franchises available in London - news and information and a general entertainment service. The London news franchise was awarded to London Broadcasting Company (LBC) and they began broadcasting on October 8th 1973. Capital Radio was awarded the general entertainment contract and their first broadcast took place eight days later. The Glasgow contract was won by Radio Clyde who made their debut on New Years Evc 1973.

Altogether, 19 contracts were awarded between 1973 and 1976. The development of ILR paused at this point as the Labour Party had been returned to power. The Labour government was wary of commercial organisations running radio stations and so temporarily halted any further development of the Independent Local Radio system.

Surprisingly, a part of the British Isles had already experienced commercial radio nearly a decade earlier. In 1959, The Tynwald, the government of The Isle Of Man, passed a bill to establish an independent commercially funded radio station on the island. They thought that a radio station would greatly benefit the community and the economy. Although the Isle of Man is self-governing, The Tynwald was required to apply to the UK authorities for a transmitting licence. The British government opposed the project but eventually the necessary permissions were granted.

The station went on air using an FM frequency of 89.0 MHz in June 1964. The first broadcast was a commentary about the Isle of Man TT race. They transmitted from studios in a caravan just outside Douglas with a temporary aerial mast located next to the caravan. In October a medium wave transmitter was established on 188 meters (1594 kHz) using a mast at Foxdale. The temporary FM mast was soon replaced with a permanent installation on Snaefell. A relay station on 91.2 MHz was added to improve reception in Douglas in 1969.

In 1965, the station moved to permanent studios on the Douglas seafront, additionally a second medium wavelength of 232 meters (1295 kHz) was allocated to improve the coverage, which had been limited by the high frequency of the 188 meters (1595 kHz) service, however the 232m service could only be used during daylight hours, so listeners had to re-tune to 188 meters when darkness fell. The programmes from Manx Radio were not only popular on the island but also with listeners across the sea in Northern Britain.

On November 23rd 1978, there was a comprehensive re-organisation of medium and long wave frequencies. These changes were intended to make more efficient use of frequencies and to reduce interference. All medium wave stations were re-aligned into strict 9kHz spacing, for local BBC and ILR stations this was just a case of altering frequency by one or two kilohertz, for example Capital Radio moved from 1546 to 1548 kHz while LBC and Clyde moved from 1151 to 1152 kHz. One exception was Manx Radio on the Isle of Man, which had its day and night time frequencies of 1295 and 1594 kHz replaced by one frequency of 1368 kHz, which would be used around the clock.

The big changes in the UK were for BBC national radio. The BBC World Service and Radio Four vacated their frequencies leaving

Radio One free to transfer to 275 and 285 metres (1089 and 1053 kHz). The pop music network also benefited from a network of much more powerful transmitters. Radio Three lost the 647 kHz signal from Daventry and moved to Radio One's old slot on 247 metres (1214 kHz), which suffered co-channel interference in many parts of the country. The 648 kHz channel was re-allocated to the BBC World Service, and was transmitted to Europe from the Orfordness transmitting station. Radio Four left medium wave and transferred to Long Wave 198 kHz. Radio Two in turn left 200 kHz long wave and moved to two of the old Radio Four wavelengths - 433 & 330 metres (693 and 909 kHz). This move paved the way for Radio Two to broadcast around the clock in January 1979.

Radio Four's move to a being a fully national service on long wave meant that spare frequencies were available. The BBC seized the opportunity to introduce Radio Scotland and Radio Wales as totally separate networks. Up to this point, listeners in Scotland and Wales heard opt out programming from Radio Four.

In 1979, the Conservative government led by Margaret Thatcher swept to power and the expansion of the Independent Local Radio network resumed. A second block of ILR franchises were issued between 1980 and 1984. Radio Mercury was the last of the original stations to go on air. Their opening broadcast was transmitted on October 20th 1984.

Despite this ruling there were a few casualties along the way. Centre Radio went into receivership on October 6th 1983 and in Wales, CBC combined with Gwent Broadcasting to become Red Dragon Radio. This entity became a much more successful venture. In 1985, Radio West in Bristol merged with Wiltshire Radio and was renamed GWR. A decade later, GWR would introduce network programming and revolutionise British local radio forever.

However, despite these setbacks, the expansion of local radio didn't stop there. In 1986 the IBA sanctioned the idea that different services could be broadcast on each station's FM and AM frequency. To test the situation, the IBA and the Home Office set up a two-year experiment. Selected stations were asked to produce different programming simultaneously on the AM and FM frequencies.

Marcher Sound provided separate programming in Welsh and the Radio Trent Group vastly expanded its Asian programming. The Asian programme Sabras moved from five hours on two days to 16 hours across seven. Meanwhile Viking Radio offered their listeners a choice of rugby league or country music. Piccadilly Radio broadcast the Halle Proms live and Capital Radio trialled CFM, a special service featuring adult oriented rock.

These experimental split frequency broadcasts were declared a big success. In 1988 the government effectively declared the end of simulcasting. They issued a decree that meant ILR stations had to provide different programming on each of their wavebands. If they failed to do this they would forfeit permission to broadcast on both FM and AM.

The first station to permanently split their frequencies was Guildford's County Sound who re-branded the FM output as Premier Radio and turned the AM output into a new golden oldies station, County Sound Gold in 1988. Other stations swiftly followed suit.

In addition to the ever-expanding list of official stations, there continued to be some illegal alternatives. Despite the efforts of the authorities, pirates are alive and well with several stations regularly on the air around the country. However, unlike their watery predecessors, these unlicensed operations were firmly land-based. Also the individuals behind these stations were not businessmen hoping to make money. Instead, early stations such as Radio Free London, Radio Jackie and Kaleidoscope were run by disgruntled fans of offshore radio that were unhappy with the official alternatives.

These early land-based stations proliferated in several major conurbations and broadcast mainly on medium wave. All of the programming was pre-recorded and transmitted from a remote area. They would string up a wire aerial between tall objects such as trees or lampposts. Then attach a cassette player to a home made transmitter powered by a car battery. This primitive set up was highly effective and could generate a good signal that propagated over a wide area.

These land-based pirates established a strong foothold in the London area during the late '60s and early '70s and got more sophisticated as time went on. Radio Jackie was really a 'community' radio station and campaigned vigorously for a licence to broadcast in their native South West London. They did have a year or so of actual live round the clock broadcasting but eventually closed down after a particularly heavy raid by the Home Office in 1985.

Eventually the pirates began to move away from being offshore tribute stations. Instead they began to target a niche audience of music fans who felt ignored by mainstream radio. Broadcasting mainly from tower blocks, these onshore pirates were the pioneers of the pirate scene that exists today. These stations thrived during the 80s playing mainly reggae and soul music. At their height there were more than 50 stations broadcasting to London including Invicta 94.2, Horizon, LWR and Solar.

The Government introduced tough new legislation in December 1988 and a lot of the original land-based pirates closed down. However a third generation of pirates such as Sunrise, Centreforce, Fantasy 98.1, and Dance FM gradually replaced them. This coincided with the emergence of dance music as a major influence in the UK. With the rise of house, hardcore and later drum & bass, a fourth generation of pirates like Dream, Kool FM, Rush and Pulse FM took control of the London airwaves. BBC Radio One has also recognised the importance of the dance scene and recruited many former pirate DJ's to front their specialist output.

A couple of prates have successfully made the transition to fully licensed stations. During its unofficial period, Kiss FM claimed a massive half a million listeners with its mix of soul, house and hip-hop. The station closed down in 1988 with the goal of obtaining an official licence. Kiss FM eventually succeeded and was granted a licence in September 1990 on its second attempt.

Radio Jackie, the early pirate pioneer, applied for a regional licence when one became available for their area in 1996. However the new FM licence was awarded to Thames Radio instead. After a few years Thames Radio experienced financial problems and the station was put up for sale The original Jackie management team swooped to purchase the loss-making station, which was relaunched as Radio Jackie on Sunday October 19th 2003.

The implementation of the 1990 Broadcasting Act led to several major radio developments for the BBC and commercial radio sectors. The government launched a radio spectrum audit and decreed that the BBC would have to end simulcasting its services on both AM and FM frequencies. This meant that the BBC would relinquish some AM frequencies and Radio One and Radio Two would broadcast on FM only. However the execution of this policy meant that a number of programmes, which were previously broadcast as opt-outs on one frequency only, would otherwise have been left without a home.

So the BBC introduced Radio Five which began at 9am on August 27th 1990. The new network broadcast on the old Radio Two AM frequencies of 693 and 909 kHz. The first voice heard on the station belonged to a five year old boy called Andrew Kelly who uttered the words "Good morning and welcome to Radio Five". There followed a prerecorded programme called 'Take Five' introduced by Bruno Brookes. Many local broadcasters received their first national exposure on the network. Local radio stalwarts like Danny Baker, Mark Radcliffe, Martin Kelner and Mark Lamarr all made their national debut on Radio Five.

Broadcasting for around 18 hours per day, the new network was to transmit a variety of sports, children's, educational and minority interest programmes. However Radio Five was not a ratings success due to its very uneven programme mix. Many saw the station as broadcasting programming the other four main BBC stations didn't want. Even the BBC's Director General at the time criticised it openly. John Birt said that Radio Five sounded "improvised and disjointed".

In January 1991, Operation Desert Storm was launched, in response to the Iraqi invasion of Kuwait. Radio Four's FM frequencies were used to provide an all-news network for the coverage of the war. 'Radio Four News FM' was well received and the positive response to the rolling news format prompted the BBC to look into the possibility of providing a full-time news station. It was decided that Radio Five would relaunch as a combined news and sport channel. The "old" Radio 5 signed off at midnight on Sunday March 27th 1994 and the new Radio Five Live began its 24-hour service at 5 am the following day.

Perhaps the biggest development to come from the 1990 Broadcasting Act was the abolition of the IBA and the introduction of a new regulator. The Radio Authority had a different remit to its predecessor. It would be allowed to issue licences to the highest bidder and promote the development of commercial radio choice.

This led to the awarding of three national contracts for Independent National Radio.

INR1 was the only one of the three new franchises that would broadcast on FM. This franchise was advertised as a non-pop licence, and was awarded to Classic FM, which launched on September 7th 1992. Classic FM enjoyed almost instantaneous success, providing listeners with a quality programme of 'accessible' classical and orchestral music and a comprehensive news service.

The other two franchises would not fare so well. INR2 was allocated the former medium wave frequency of BBC Radio Three. This licence was awarded to Virgin 1215 with a service of rock-orientated music. The new service began on April 30th 1993 and was popular amongst rock fans. However Virgin was not the financial success a national music station could have been and the adventurous music policy was increasingly diluted and became more conventional. The station has since become Absolute Radio and utilised new broadcasting technologies to launch several complementary digital services.

The Radio Authority awarded the third franchise to Talk Radio UK, which started transmissions on Valentines Day in 1995. The station utilised the old Radio One AM outlets vacated by the BBC's pop network in 1994. At its launch, the station employed many 'shock jocks' whose aim was to provoke debate by being deliberately outrageous. However this American style of presentation proved to be unpopular with British audiences and prompted the station to alter the format fairly swiftly. The confrontational approach of presentation was replaced by more traditional 'phone-in' shows. Talk Radio UK employed experienced speech presenters such as James Whale, Mike Allen, Paul Ross, Mike Dickin and Nick Abbot.

Despite gaining a fairly sizeable audience, Talk Radio seemed unable to generate a profit. In 1999, the station was taken over by The Wireless Group in partnership with media mogul Rupert Murdoch. The station re-launched as 'TalkSport' with former newspaper editor Kelvin Mackenzie at the helm. Under his leadership the station enjoyed a renaissance - audiences increased considerably and this led to the station becoming profitable. In 2005 The Wireless Group was sold to Ulster Television and TalkSport became part of UTV Radio.

The Radio Authority began to licence low-power temporary radio stations for special events, operating for up to 28 days a year. They also reduced the criteria for a "viable service area" with the introduction of small scale local licences for towns, villages and special interest groups.

At this point in time the AM waveband had become unpopular with radio groups and the majority of new stations were awarded an FM licence only, even when an AM licence was jointly available. The Radio Authority also introduced regional stations and began to licence the commercial Digital Audio Broadcasting (DAB) multiplexes in October 1998.

The Radio Authority's lighter touch also meant a relaxation of ownership rules. Tentatively stations began to form small local groups to take advantage of the financial opportunities this produced. Stations in the group could share news and sales operations. Gradually, several distinct large radio groups evolved. These included EMAP (Now Bauer) and The Wireless Group (Now UTV). Capital Radio merged with the GWR group in 2005 to form Gcap Media plc (now owned by Global Radio).

As these acquisitions and mergers gathered pace, specialist local programmes were dropped and output began being shared around the networks. Most of the localised medium wave 'gold' or 'classic hits' stations disappeared and became either 'Capital Gold', 'Classic Gold' or 'Magic'. The networking of programmes would proliferate rapidly and would not just be confined to medium wave outlets.

Even with the best of intentions, existing radio services can't hope to cater for the full range of listeners' interests. Special interest material will always be marginalised in a mainstream schedule. The homogenised output of the radio networks has left many listeners disenfranchised and this led to many groups calling for a third tier of radio broadcasting to be introduced.

There were two distinct factions promoting this third tier. Firstly, there were those who desired a simple deregulation of the airwaves. When this happened in France and Italy it led to even more similar sounding stations being introduced and a lack of real choice for the listener. The groups seeking deregulation have been largely ignored by the authorities in favour of the second faction – individuals or ethnic groups seeking to introduce community radio to their area.

The meaning of community radio is straightforward: It is radio that is owned, managed and made by its audience. Any member of the public can become a member of the group running their local station and make and broadcast programmes, without being filtered through the mediating hands of the professionals.

Community radio stations were in operation on cable systems as far back as 1978. In the late 80s the then newly formed Radio Authority awarded licences (termed "Incremental" by the outgoing Independent Broadcasting Authority) to a number of new, ex-pirate and cable based community ventures. These stations were introduced to provide extra specialist stations for areas with an existing commercial radio station.

The first four incremental stations were granted licences in 1989. They were Sunset 102 in Manchester, CentreSound in Stirling, FTP in Bristol and Sunrise Radio in West London. They were forbidden to seek public funding and advertising was their only source of income. Not surprisingly many of these new stations crashed and burned very quickly. FTP and CentreSound failed within a year of launching and, after a managerial restructure, were relaunched as Galaxy 97.2 and Central FM respectively. Sunset Radio lasted until October 1993 before filing for bankruptcy. Faze FM were awarded the re-advertised 102.0 FM licence and operated under the name Kiss 102. Rather than a community station, Kiss was a dance music station and was later sold to Galaxy Radio.

The only one of the first four to survive intact was Sunrise Radio. Sunrise quickly expanded, first into Bradford, taking over the licence for the failed Bradford Community Radio. A satellite service followed in 1991. Then in 1994, Sunrise Radio won the Radio Authority licensing process to expand its programming across the whole of London and the surrounding counties from the 50kW transmitter at Brookman's Park.

Some other stations have survived and thrived. Spectrum Radio, a multi ethnic foreign language station serving greater London on 558 kHz medium wave has been a successful project and remains on air. Another London station served a specialist interest group rather than a minority ethnic audience. London Jazz Radio launched as Jazz FM with a professional team of presenters and a signal similar to Capital Radio.

For a while things seemed to be going well, the organization also won the North West of England regional licence. However Jazz FM could never make enough money to be sustainable in that form. The station's name was changed to JFM in an effort to re-brand but the Jazz FM name was re-instated a few years later. Jazz FM was eventually purchased by GMG Media who changed the format to oldies and tuneful pop and renamed it Smooth Radio. Jazz FM was re-launched in 2008 as an on-line and digital station.

Many other incremental stations were unsuccessful. RWL (Radio West Lothian) 1368, which was based in Bathgate, failed very quickly in 1990. East End Radio in Glasgow lost its licence several years after going on air. Radio Harmony, the ethnic station in Coventry, remained on air for several years before being taken over by KIX-96, a mainstream pop music station. It was a similar story with Belfast Community Radio (BCR) that, after six years of struggling, flipped to a mainstream pop format in 1996.

Radio managed to retain a sizeable audience during the last half of the 20th century despite the rising dominance of television. It did this by constantly evolving and adapting to audience needs and economic trends. However as the new millennium began, radio would face stiff competition from even more emerging technologies.

11

Radio in the 21st Century

At the beginning of the 21st century there was a radical shift in how listeners received music and information. Young people in particular saw radio as outmoded. They preferred to listen to music or access news and information via portable music players and the Internet.

There has been a noticeable drift away from AM to FM broadcasts since the new century began. Audiences for long, medium and short wave broadcasts continue to fall. In fact many international broadcasters have ceased their short wave transmissions and increasingly the only things that can be heard on this band are radio hams, utility and time stations.

However this doesn't mean that radio has finally been eclipsed. Radio simply did what it did when confronted by the emergence of television in the 1950s – adapt to survive. Radio moved from being a linear broadcast on one device to unique audio content delivered via multiple platforms. Emerging technologies such as satellite, digital broadcasting and the Internet offered radio stations a multi-platform future. As digital forms of radio proliferate, listeners will enjoy an abundance of new programming.

Radio has fought off competition from broadband Internet, YouTube, Spotify or Facebook. Indeed, its strength is that you can still enjoy radio while you do many of these things. Podcasts or 'listen on demand' facilities on radio station websites are enabling audiences who didn't catch the original broadcast to listen later at a time that suits them.

RAJAR figures in 2010 showed that the number of people listening to radio on these new platforms is still quite small. Live radio through the TV accounts for just 4.3% of total radio listening. Radio through the Internet is even lower, at just 3.1%.

Many traditional radio stations now have an outlet on the Internet. Internet radio utilises streaming media, presenting listeners with a continuous stream of audio that cannot be paused or replayed. Streaming on the Internet is usually referred to as webcasting since it's not transmitted using traditional broadcast methods. Internet

Radio is distinct from on-demand file serving and podcasting, which involves downloading the material rather than streaming.

It's highly disputed as to who first thought of Internet radio but records show that the first actual Internet radio station was by a non-profit organization called The Internet Multi-casting Company of Washington, which began in 1993. On November 7th 1994, WXYC in North Carolina became the first traditional radio station to announce broadcasting on the Internet. They were joined a week later by WREK in Atlanta. These stations used their own streaming software but Progressive Networks released RealAudio in 1995. This software took advantage of the latest advances in digital compression and delivered AM radio-quality sound in real time. Eventually, companies such as Nullsoft and Microsoft released their own streaming audio players and many web-based radio stations began to proliferate.

In March 1996, Virgin Radio became the first European radio station to broadcast its full schedule live on the Internet. It broadcast its FM signal, live from the source, simultaneously on the Internet 24 hours a day. Nowadays even small community and hospital stations have an Internet stream and can subsequently be heard well outside of their locality.

As DSL and Broadband Internet replaced the old dial-up phone line connections, Internet radio became more popular. Undoubtedly broadcast radio remains the best way to reach hundreds of thousands of people at the same time. Despite this, many people believe that the Internet will become the main delivery method for radio in the future. It seems difficult to understand their reasoning, as webcasting could be an impossibly costly broadcast medium for both radio broadcasters and listeners.

Let's take the broadcasters first. The station has to allocate space on a server for each online listener. The more listeners a radio station has – the more expensive it becomes. It could also prove highly expensive for a listener who wants to listen to an Internet radio stream while on the move. In America, 50% of total listening hours are spent in a mobile situation, such as a car. In the UK, the figures are somewhat lower at around 25%. Radio via a mobile phone would never be able to replace broadcast radio in terms of technical quality: the coverage levels simply aren't adequate in most parts of the world. Also mobile phone operators are beginning to limit their customer's data usage and listening to a radio station via a 3G smartphone would swiftly eat up their monthly data allowance

In 2004, radio in Britain fell under the control of the Office of Communications, commonly known as Ofcom. This new regulator also replaced the Independent Television Commission, the Broadcasting Standards Council, the Radio Communications Agency and the Office of Telecommunications.

In addition to AM and FM transmission methods, radio stations gained a digital alternative. The Broadcasting Act of 1996 allowed the introduction of national, regional and local Digital Broadcasting to Britain. Traditional broadcasting methods used up a comparatively large amount of spectrum for a relatively small number of stations. Digital Audio Broadcasting (DAB) combines multiple audio streams onto a relatively narrow band centred on a single broadcast frequency called a DAB ensemble or multiplex.

The BBC had started digital radio test transmissions from Crystal Palace as far back as 1990 and permanent transmissions to London began in September 1995. With the expansion of its network in the spring of 1998, the BBC's digital radio ensemble was available to 65% of the UK population by 2001 and to 85% by 2004.

All the BBC's existing radio services appeared on the digital ensemble, including the World Service. This was the first time the station was available to a domestic audience in crystal clear quality. However there were more digital delights to come.

The arrival of five new digital services in 2002 marked the largest expansion of radio in the BBC's history. 5 Live Sports Extra, a companion station to 5 Live, was the first to launch in February of that year The part time station provided uninterrupted sports coverage when there were clashes of major events where the BBC had the broadcasting rights.

6 Music, the BBC's first new national music station for 32 years, followed in March 2002. This station filled the gap between Radios One and Two, offering an alternative mix of classic and contemporary rock music. In addition, other specialist genres such as jazz, funk, blues and folk would also be featured. The BBC's vast archives of live music sessions would form an important part of 6 Music's programmes.

1Xtra, a sister station to Radio One was launched on August 16th 2002. This station was aimed at young fans of cutting edge urban music, such as rap, hip-hop and R&B. As well as contemporary black music, the station featured a dedicated news service and regular speech-based programmes.

The BBC Asian Network, already a successful regional service on FM in the West Midlands and the North, launched nationwide on October 28th 2002. Offering a mix of news and music, this station was aimed at the diverse Asian communities across the UK. The station broadcasts mainly in English, but also features programmes in various south Asian languages – Hindi, Urdu, Punjabi, Bengali, Gujurati and the Mirpuri dialect of the Potwari language.

BBC 7, a new speech station, was launched in December 2002. This station was the principal broadcasting outlet for the BBC's archive of spoken-word entertainment and many old favourites like Hancock's Half Hour and Dick Barton were rebroadcast to a modern audience. The station was rebranded as BBC Radio 4 Extra on April 2nd 2011 to bring the station closer to its sister station, Radio Four.

The first national licence for DAB from the Radio Authority was advertised in 1998 and only one applicant applied. The licence was awarded to the GWR Group and NTL Broadcast. The two companies formed the Digital One multiplex, which began broadcasting on 15 November 1999. The Digital One multiplex has grown and is currently available to over 90% of the UK population. The United Kingdom presently has the world's biggest digital radio network, with 103 transmitters, two national ensembles and 48 local and regional ensembles broadcasting over 250 commercial and 34 BBC radio stations.

Despite the existence of the DAB network, the medium initially struggled to gain mass acceptance by consumers. Cost was a major issue in the early days. Digital radios were first sold as car radios in 1997, priced around £800. Hi-fi tuners costing up to £2,000 were released two years later. In 2002, Pure Digital's Evoke series of radios broke the £100 price barrier and the cost of a digital radio has since fallen to around £40.

Lower prices, new radio stations and marketing have increased the uptake of DAB radio in the UK Nowadays it's estimated that 32% of the population possesses a DAB digital radio set. RAJAR, who measure radio listening figures in the UK, stated in March 2011 that 26.5% of radio listening in the UK is done through digital platforms at least once a week. 16.7% of digital radio listening was to digital only stations and 4.1% of digital radio users listen to digital radio through a television platform. Electrical retailer Dixon's announced in 2006 that it would discontinue selling analogue radios.

DAB was promoted in Britain as having two major advantages over analogue radio broadcasting in that using compression technology, parts of the audio spectrum that cannot be heard by humans are discarded, meaning less data needs to be sent over the air. This, as well as multiplexing technology, allows a number of channels to be broadcast together on one frequency as opposed to one channel for analogue radio broadcasts. This meant that broadcasters were able to launch exclusive digital radio stations alongside their existing analogue stations. Broadcasters also state that DAB offers better reception and is resistant to the interference which other broadcast media are susceptible to. DAB radios also come with additional features such as scrolling text, providing information such as breaking news, travel information or the latest track information.

However DAB's critics say that the audio quality on DAB is lower than on FM. 98% of stereo stations use a bit rate level of 128kbs with the MP2 audio codec. A bit rate of 256kbs would be required to achieve a 'CD quality' signal. Also, a large and growing number of music stations are transmitting in mono. Indeed, the bit rates used by the radio stations on other digital platforms, such as cable, terrestrial and satellite are usually higher than on DAB, so the audio quality is also higher. On the other hand, an Ofcom survey, which was undertaken due to many consultation responses citing poor DAB quality, found that 94% of DAB listeners thought DAB was at least as good as FM.

Also some areas of the country are not presently covered by DAB; the BBC says that it may not be able to provide coverage to the final 10% of the population, and may use DRM instead. Ofcom estimate that even after extra spectrum has been allocated to DAB, around 90 local radio stations will be unable to transmit on DAB, either because there is no space for them on a local DAB multiplex, or because they cannot afford the high transmission costs of DAB that the multiplex operators are charging.

The United Kingdom Government intends to migrate the vast majority of AM and FM analogue services to digital in 2015, subject to targets being met for coverage and listening figures for digital radio. However ministers are currently considering pushing the switchover back to 2017 at the earliest.

WorldDMB, the organisation in charge of the DAB standards, announced DAB+, a major upgrade to the DAB standard in 2006. The new standard is not backward compatible so older receivers cannot receive DAB+ broadcasts. DAB+ broadcasts have launched in several countries like Switzerland, Malta, Italy and Australia and several other countries are also expected to launch DAB+ broadcasts over the next few years.

The USA adopted a different digital technology to that of Europe. HD Radio, which originally stood for "Hybrid Digital", was the method selected by the Federal Communications Commission in 2002. HD is an in-band on-channel, or IBOC, digital radio technology. It's used by AM and FM radio stations to transmit audio and data via a digital signal in conjunction with their analogue signals. While HD Radio does allow for an all-digital mode, this system currently is used by some AM and FM radio stations to simulcast both digital and analogue audio within the same channel as well as to add new FM channels and text information.

Although HD Radio broadcasting's content is currently subscription-free, listeners must purchase new receivers in order to receive the digital portion of the signal. In May 2009, there were more stations in the world on the air with HD Radio technology than any other digital radio technology. More than 1,900 stations covering approximately 84% of the United States were broadcasting with this technology, and more than 1,000 additional HD2 and HD3 multicast channels were on the air.

The USA doesn't intend to force off analogue radio broadcasts as it has with analogue television broadcasts, as it would not result in the recovery of any radio spectrum rights which could be sold. Therefore there is no deadline by which consumers must buy an HD Radio receiver. In addition, there are many more analogue AM/FM radio receivers than there were analogue televisions, and many of these are car stereos or portable units that cannot be upgraded.

Another way of relaying high quality broadcasts is via satellite. In Europe many radio stations provide an additional broadcast outlet via the Astra satellite. Using this facility, local and national stations can reach far beyond their country's boundaries. All the BBC radio channels are available via Sky or Freesat. Radio services on these platforms are generally free to air but there are some radio services that are subscription-based. These are generally digital packages of numerous channels that don't broadcast terrestrially, most notably in North America.

Some of these services, such as Music Choice or Muzak, require a fixed-location receiver and a dish antenna. Launched in 1987, Music Choice was the first digital audio broadcast service in the world. The organisation produces music-related content for digital cable, cell phones, and cable modem subscribers in the United States.

Mobile satellite services, such as Sirius, XM, and Worldspace, offered listeners the chance to travel across an entire continent, listening to the same audio programming anywhere they go. Sirius was the first to begin broadcasting on January 5th 2001. Tim McGraw was the first artist ever played on satellite radio. He gave a special welcome introduction which segued into his song "Things Change".

XM uses fixed-location geostationary satellites in two positions to beam their signals down to earth. Sirius uses three geosynchronous satellites in highly elliptical orbits passing over North and South America, to transmit the digital streams. The Sirius signal comes from a high elevation angle in the northern part of the continent. This higher angle makes the signal less vulnerable to drop out in cities, but more likely to disappear in tunnels and other covered areas. In these cases local signal boosters are required.

Worldspace operated from Silver Spring, Maryland with additional studios located in Washington D.C., Bangalore, Mumbai, New Delhi, and Nairobi. The company employed two satellites and broadcast 62 channels - 38 of which were content provided by international, national and regional third parties. At its height, Worldspace had over 170,000 subscribers in Eastern and Southern Africa, the Middle East, and Asia.

However mobile satellite services have proved difficult to sustain. Worldspace filed for bankruptcy in 2008 and European operations were liquidated the following spring. Sirius and XM only survived after the companies merged in July 2008.

Listening to radio on additional platforms such as satellite and the Internet will steadily increase. However broadcast radio will continue to be the predominant medium through which we enjoy radio.

We heard previously that the early community radio experiment, which started in Britain in the early 1990s, had largely failed. With a few notable exceptions, the initial incremental stations were not able to survive because of commercial pressures. Undaunted, the community radio sector lobbied successive governments to introduce a third tier of broadcasting.

In 2002, the Radio Authority licensed fifteen 'Access Radio stations' for a trial period of one year to test the feasibility of such stations. These pilot stations targeted a wide range of minorities and groups. Angel Radio in Hampshire targeted the over-60s while Awaz FM was aimed at the Asian population in Glasgow. Resonance FM served the artistic community in London while Takeover Radio gave the children of Leicester their own radio station. All the licenses were extended in 2003 for another year.

The Community Radio Order 2004 established the final legal framework for full-time, long-term community radio licences in the UK. Community radio services are operated on a not-for-profit basis with community ownership and control built in to their structures. To obtain a community radio licence, applicants must demonstrate that the proposed station will meet the needs of a specified target community, together with required "social gain" objectives set out in the application. These usually take the form of a commitment to train local people in broadcasting skills or provide a certain amount of programming aimed at an underserved section of the population.

Following pressure from the UK's Commercial Radio Companies Association, community radio stations are subject to varying funding stipulations based on a community radio station's proximity to a commercial radio broadcaster. No community radio station is permitted to raise more than 50% of its operating costs from a single source, including on-air sponsorship and advertising. The remainder of operating costs must be met through other sources such as grants, donor income, National Lottery funding or charities. However, where a community radio station lies totally within the transmission area of a commercial station with a population of 150,000 or less, no sponsorship or advertising is permitted and all funding must come from alternative sources. In a small number of areas a community radio station may not be licensed at all. This is to protect the financial interests of smaller commercial stations.

There was a second round of licensing in 2007, followed by third in 2011. To date over 228 licences have been granted. However it has not been an unqualified success. Several community stations have closed down due to lack of funds or resources. These included three of the original pilot stations – Forest of Dean Radio in Gloucestershire, Sound Radio in Hackney and Northern Visions Radio in Belfast.

The broadcast regulator Ofcom would preside over radio during a turbulent period for the industry. A financial downturn and a relaxation of the programming rules meant that a number of established radio stations disappeared. Quasi-national networks replaced these stations. Familiar names such as Beacon Radio, Leicester Sound, and Mercia FM were re branded as Heart, Smooth or Capital.

These networks are controlled, programmed and run from one location (usually London) with the facility to opt out locally for news and advertisements. These homogeneous stations tend to air just a few hours of locally originated programmes per day and then switch over to the network output. At network centre, the presenters there have the facility to record different links for each location, which are then transmitted, by the individual station. The average listener could be quite oblivious to the fact that their local transmissions are in fact emanating from a studio hundreds of miles away.

A significant amount of listeners were outraged that their local stations were axed and replaced by the networked output. However for the big radio groups, there are sound economic reasons for networking programmes from a central source - the most obvious ones being reduced staffing and administration costs. So far the decision seems to have paid off as audience figures have remained at the levels they were before the introduction of networking. In some cases the audience has increased.

In North America, the dissemination of programming from a distant source is nothing new. The syndication of programmes has been widespread for decades. Before radio networks matured in the United States, some early radio shows were reproduced on transcription disks and mailed to individual stations.

An early example of syndication using this method was RadiOzark Enterprises, Inc. based in Springfield, Missouri. The company produced a half-hour programme called 'Sermons in Song' and distributed it to 200 stations in the 1940s. RadiOzark later produced country music shows starring Tennessee Ernie Ford Smiley Burnette, and George Morgan.

Many syndicated radio programmes were distributed by post, although the medium changed as technology developed, going from transcription disks to vinyl records, tape recordings and CDs. Since the advent of the Internet, many stations have opted to distribute programmes via CD-quality MP3s. Nowadays most live syndicated radio shows are distributed using satellite sub carrier audio technology.

The Telecommunications Act of 1996, which led to significant concentration of media ownership, facilitated the rapid deployment of both existing and new syndicated programs in the late 1990s, putting syndication on par with, and eventually surpassing, the network radio format.

Radio syndication generally works the same way as television syndication, except that radio stations usually are not organized into strict affiliate-only networks. Nowadays radio networks generally are only distributors of radio shows, and individual stations can decide which shows to carry from a wide variety of networks and independent sources.

Some examples of widely syndicated music programmes include 'Rick Dees' Weekly Top 40' and the nightly request programme, 'Delilah', heard on many U.S. stations. Syndication is particularly popular in talk radio. Most talk radio stations are free to assemble their own lineup of hosts like Sean Hannity, Jim Bohannon, Rush Limbaugh and Don Imus.

National Public Radio, American Public Media and Public Radio International all supply programmes to local public radio member stations. Some radio shows are also offered on a barter system usually at no charge to the radio station. The system is used for live programming or preproduced programs and includes a mixture of ad time sold by the programme producer as well as time set aside for the radio station to sell.

American radio continues to innovate. Smart media analysts continue to pay close attention to the American radio scene as it usually provides an indication of trends to come. Where America leads the rest of the world soon follows.

And that brings us to the present day. Despite the technological, cultural and economic shifts of the 21st century radio continues to thrive. Television or the Internet may have become the main way the general public consume their media but radio continues to be a valuable asset. Radio doesn't need to drastically change its core characteristics. Its simplicity and portability will ensure it remains.

What radio does need to do is continue its progress into a digital world. It needs to pay close attention to the changing pattern of consumer and listener behaviour. Radio needs to seek out new markets and continue to innovate and adapt to new technology. By adopting new broadcast platforms such as satellite, digital or the Internet, radio faces a multi-platform future. Radio will continue to occupy an important place in the media landscape of the 21st century.

BIBLIOGRAPHY

The Early History of Radio: From Faraday to Marconi - G. R. M. Garratt

Days Seemed Longer – Roy Plomley

The Birth of Broadcasting: The History of Broadcasting in the United Kingdom - Asa Briggs

Laughter in the Air: An Informal History of British Radio Comedy – Barry Took

Scotland on the Air – George Burnett

On My Wavelength – Howard Lockhart

The Golden Age of Radio: An Illustrated Companion – Dennis Gifford

A Concise History of British Radio 1922 – 1982 – Sean Street

The History of BBC Broadcasting in Scotland 1923-1983 - W H McDowell

Under The Bedclothes – Janet Alldis

The Emergence of Broadcasting in Britain – Brian Hennessey

The Radio Companion – Paul Donovan

Pop Went the Pirates: History of Offshore Radio Stations – Keith Skues

And The World Listened: The Story of Captain Leonard Frank Plugge – Keith Willis

Those Radio Times – Susan Briggs

208 It Was Great – Alan Bailey

American Radio Networks: A History – Jim Cox

Wireless Radio: A Brief History – Lewis Coe

Crossing the Ether – Sean Street

Radio Luxembourg the Station of the Stars – Richard Nichols

Radio Goes To War – Gerd Horten